Heal Endometriosis

Dr. Susan's Healthy Living
drsusanshealthyliving.com

Facebook.com/DrSusanRichards
drsusanshealthyliving@gmail.com
(650) 561-9978

Mention of specific companies or products in this book does not suggest endorsement by the author or publisher. Internet addresses and telephone numbers for resources provided in this book were accurate at the time it went to press.

ISBN 978-1511974950

Note

The information in this book is meant to complement the advice and guidance of your physician, not replace it. It is very important that any person who has medical problems be evaluated by a physician. If you are under the care of a physician, you should discuss any major changes in your regimen with him or her. Because this is a book and not a medical consultation, keep in mind that the information presented here may not apply in your particular case. In view of individual medical requirements, new research, and government regulations, it is the responsibility of the reader to validate health practices and treatments with a physician or health service.

Table of Contents

Introduction

Dear Friend,

I am thrilled that you have found my book, **Heal Endometriosis**, because I know that you are looking for positive and effective all-natural solutions to deal with this issue and bring your symptoms under control. I know how difficult and debilitating this problem is since I have successfully treated thousands of patients with endometriosis in my clinical practice. I have written this book just for you, to share with you my all-natural treatment program that has helped so many of my patients recover from this painful condition.

I have always loved working with my patients as a team effort and it has reaped great results! It has been very gratifying and heartwarming to see so many women regain their hormonal health with my program. I hope that this information is helpful for you, too.

Endometriosis is a hormone-related inflammatory condition that causes painful implants and scarring in a woman's pelvis. This potentially devastating condition affects millions of women during their prime reproductive years, most often from their twenties through their early fifties and even beyond into menopause. These are the years when women are starting to develop their careers and families – a time of new and exciting life experiences. Energy and a zest for life are often at their peak.

If you are like the millions of women who suffer from endometriosis, I know that this condition has probably affected the quality of your life. Perhaps you are suffering from menstrual pain and cramping or heavy menstrual bleeding. Many of my patients have come to me with symptoms that were initially so intense that their ability to work, care for children, enjoy personal relationships, have all been affected. Endometriosis has even affected their ability to engage in sexual intercourse during a period of several days to several weeks each month. Endometriosis is also a common cause of infertility and can affect the ability of some women to bear children.

Endometriosis is often triggered by high levels of estrogen (estrogen dominance) as well as by painful inflammation. Stress and nutritional factors can also play major roles in this problem. Women with moderate to severe endometriosis are often treated with many different drug and hormonal therapies that only control their symptoms for a short period of time and often have significant side effects. In addition, many of these women face a high risk of eventually having a hysterectomy.

Happily, my all-natural treatment program has been very successful in relieving the painful symptoms of this conditions and even sparing many of my patients from having to undergo hysterectomy. Unlike medication and surgery, which seeks to control the symptoms of this condition, my program has been developed to actually correct the hormonal and chemical imbalances that have triggered this condition in the first place. Thus, the correction is more profound and gets to the root causes of this issue. As a result, you are likely to have benefits for your entire menstrual cycle and reproductive health.

I want to share with you one of my cases: my patient Joyce, a 41 year old woman, whose symptoms of endometriosis were so severe that they drastically affected the quality of her life. Her gynecologist had even recommended a hysterectomy after medication had not halted the worsening of this condition. Joyce came to me seeking relief from her symptoms through natural therapies and wanting to avoid having a hysterectomy, if at all possible.

When Joyce and I first started to work together, she complained of severe menstrual cramping in her pelvis and abdomen as well as low back pain. She found sex difficult to engage in with her husband since she had pain on intercourse. Her menstrual periods were quite heavy and she had spotting between her periods. She had digestive symptoms during her period including bloating and diarrhea that were caused by endometriosis. In addition, she suffered from fluid retention, mood swings and irritability and food cravings for one week before each menstrual period due to PMS (premenstrual syndrome.)

I started Joyce on my all-natural endometriosis healing program. She was very motivated and eagerly followed my dietary and nutritional supplement recommendations. She also started on a stress reduction program that I created for her since her symptoms were worse during times when Joyce had more work and home stress.

Within one to two menstrual cycles, she was delighted to find that her pain and cramping as well as her PMS symptoms began to decrease very rapidly. As Joyce continued with my program, she found that her symptoms continued to improve greatly and her menstrual periods became much more comfortable. In addition, her overall quality of life was much better and, best of all, Joyce was able to avoid having a hysterectomy!

Joyce is typical of many of the women I have worked with over the years who have benefitted greatly from my all-natural endometriosis healing program. I have been thrilled to see so many of my patients recover their health and wellness from this chronic, disabling condition.

The end result of my program is not only relief from your endometriosis symptoms but also healthier and more regular menstrual periods and less premenstrual and menstrual symptoms. If you are in your forties, it will also help to ensure an easier transition into menopause with fewer symptoms! I have seen this often with my own patients. I discuss both my all-natural program as well as the medical therapies for endometriosis in great detail in this book.

My All-Natural Approach to Healing Endometriosis

My endometriosis patients have benefitted greatly by practicing the very effective program that I developed to help them gain relief from this condition. I have spent years researching the use of diet, nutrition, and many other techniques as part of a complete all-natural approach to treating this issue. I have also shared with my patients many different self-care treatment options. These therapies also help to create a healthier and better quality life. I have included all of these in this book.

I have been delighted with the positive feedback that my patients have given me. They are always pleased to find that my all-natural treatments are so beneficial and effective in relieving their symptoms.

How to Use This Book

I feel strongly that any woman interested in healing from endometriosis should have access to this information. Because there are many women whom I will never see as patients in my medical practice, I wrote this book to share the all-natural program that I have developed and found, through years of medical practice, to be most useful. I hope you will find this information as useful as my patients have. I am continuously expanding my own knowledge about the most up to date therapies and researching new healthcare techniques for treating endometriosis.

My all-natural program includes my endometriosis relief diet as well as the vitamins, minerals, essential fatty acids and herbs that I have found, are most likely to eliminate your symptoms. Utilizing a therapeutic diet and nutritional supplement program are essential to achieve endometriosis relief.

I have included the very beneficial deep breathing exercises, stress reduction techniques, acupressure massage points, stretching positions that are specifically helpful for endometriosis as well as recommendations for physical exercise. The book contains chapters on the symptoms and medical diagnosis of this condition. I also discuss the most up-to-date drug therapies and surgical procedures for endometriosis and explain the pros and cons of all of these medical treatments.

I recommend that you read through the book first to familiarize yourself with the material. The Endometriosis Workbook (Chapter 2) will help you evaluate your symptoms, your risk factors and the lifestyle habits that can affect your health. Then turn to the therapy chapters and read through the rest of the book. Try all the therapies that most appeal to you and pertain to your symptoms. Establish a regimen that works for you and follow it every day.

My endometriosis healing program is practical and easy to follow. You can use it by itself or in conjunction with a medical program. While working with a physician is necessary to establish a definitive diagnosis of this problem, and medical therapy may still be necessary for women with more severe symptoms, my all natural treatment program will help to correct and balance the hormonal and chemical imbalances that trigger this condition in the first place. For many women, this book can not only help speed up the diagnostic process but also bring you significant relief.

My all-natural treatment program can play a major role in reducing the severity of your symptoms and preventing recurrences of this condition. The feeling of wellness that can be yours with my self-care program will radiate out and touch your whole life. You will have more time and energy to enjoy your work, family, and other pleasures in life. I hope that your life is positively transformed by these beneficial therapies.

Love,

Dr. Susan

Part I:
Identifying the Problem

1

What Is Endometriosis?

I want to begin our journey together of supporting your healing from endometriosis by describing the symptoms of this condition and how it affects the organs and tissues of your body. I also discuss the risk factors that can predispose you towards developing this condition. This will help you to better understand this condition and how it is affecting your menstrual cycle as well as your health in general.

Endometriosis refers to the condition in which cells comprising the lining of the uterus, called the endometrium, break away and grow outside the uterine cavity, implanting themselves in the pelvis. These implants can occur in many locations within the pelvis, including the ovaries, ligaments of the uterus, cervix, appendix, bowel, and bladder. Occasionally, these cells can even invade distant structures such as a lung or armpit. Like the regular lining of the uterus, these implants respond to hormonal stimulation and can cause bleeding in the pelvic cavity.

Unlike normal menstrual bleeding, implant bleeding cannot leave the body through the vaginal opening during menstruation. Instead, blood from the endometrial implants remains trapped in the pelvis where it can cause inflammation, cysts, scar tissue, and other structural damage to the many tissues and organs in this area.

The endometrial implants can assume a variety of shapes and colors. They can include lesions that are tiny pinpoint areas of bleeding; white opaque plaques; or small lesions, rust or dark brown in color, that are described as "mulberry" or "raspberry" in appearance. Some medical textbooks describe these dark areas as looking like "powder burns." Fibrous tissue often grows around these lesions, giving them a puckered appearance. In more advanced cases, adhesions (scar tissue) develop around the implants. The scar tissue can be so dense that it obliterates the normal pelvic structures.

Endometrial implants on the ovary can form cysts; these cysts are often called "chocolate cysts" because they are filled with a thick, dark brown fluid that is actually old blood. The inflammatory changes, scarring, and tissue damage associated with endometrial implants can destroy and distort the normal pelvic tissues in a way that causes significant problems for affected women.

Endometriosis is considered an important gynecological problem because it can cause chronic pain and discomfort in younger women during their prime reproductive years. In fact, it is found primarily in menstruating women from age 20 to 45, with its peak incidence in the thirties and forties. It is not, however, limited to this age group; endometriosis can be found in teenagers and even occasionally in postmenopausal women, since the estrogen used in hormone replacement therapy can reactivate the endometrial implants.

Endometriosis is a relatively common problem, affecting as many as five million American women (or 7 to 15 percent of the female population). It is a major cause of chronic pain and severe menstrual cramps in younger women, affecting over 50 percent of those in their teens. The pelvic damage caused by endometriosis can also hamper childbearing. In fact, 20 to 66 percent of women with endometriosis experience infertility, a finding based on medical research and clinical studies. To better understand what causes this crippling problem, let's look at the normal menstrual cycle. This will make it easier to understand the changes in the normal process that can occur and lead to the development of endometriosis.

The Normal Menstrual Cycle

Each month women in their fertile years (before the onset of menopause, age 45 to 50) go through menstruation. Menstruation refers to the shedding of the uterine lining, or endometrium. Each month the uterus prepares a thick, blood-rich cushion to nourish and house a fertilized egg. If pregnancy doesn't occur and the egg doesn't implant in the uterus, then the body doesn't need this extra buildup of the uterine lining. The uterus cleanses itself by releasing the extra blood and tissue so that a fresh buildup can occur all over again the following month, in case a pregnancy does occur.

The mechanism that regulates the buildup and shedding of the uterine lining is controlled by fluctuations in hormonal levels. It begins each month when follicle-stimulating hormones (FSH) and luteinizing hormones (LH) are released from the pituitary, a gland located at the base of the brain. Once FSH and LH are released into the bloodstream, their destination is the ovaries. The ovaries hold all the eggs a woman will ever have, in an inactive form called follicles. During each cycle, the FSH and LH from the pituitary gland cause the follicles to ripen; normally, one egg is released for possible fertilization. As part of this process, the follicles begin to produce the hormones estrogen and progesterone. Estrogen reaches its peak during the first half of the cycle as the newly released egg is maturing. Progesterone output begins after midcycle when ovulation (the production of a mature egg cell) has occurred.

Besides preparing the egg for fertilization, estrogen and progesterone stimulate the lining of the uterus. During the first two weeks following menstruation, estrogen causes the uterine lining to gradually rebuild itself. The glands of the endometrium begin to grow long, and the lining thickens through an increase in the number of blood vessels as well as the production of a mesh of fibers that connect throughout the lining. By midcycle, the lining of the uterus has expanded three times in thickness and has a greatly increased blood supply.

After midcycle, usually around day 14, ovulation occurs. The egg is picked up by the fallopian tube and continues on to the uterus. The follicle that has produced the egg for that month (or graafian follicle) is further stimulated after midcycle by LH and changes into the yellow body, or corpus luteum. The corpus luteum secretes progesterone, which has further effects on the uterine lining, causing a coiling of the blood vessels of the endometrium. Also, the glands of the uterine lining become swollen and tortuous and secrete a thick mucous.

If the egg is fertilized, it will implant on the uterine wall and the corpus luteum will continue to secrete progesterone. If no fertilization occurs, the corpus luteum begins to deteriorate and the progesterone levels decrease. The lining of the uterus starts to break down and menstruation begins.

Besides estrogen and progesterone, the hormone-like prostaglandins also affect menstrual function by regulating the muscle tension of the uterus. Like progesterone, prostaglandin production is seen only during ovulatory menstrual cycles. Prostaglandin production increases during the second half of the cycle, peaking toward the end of the cycle with the onset of menstruation. Prostaglandins are found in many tissues in the body besides the uterus, including the gastrointestinal tract and blood vessels. All prostaglandins affect muscle tension, with some promoting smooth muscle relaxation while others trigger smooth muscle contraction.

Prostaglandins are derived from fatty acids in the diet. The series-2 prostaglandins (specifically the E2 and F2 Alpha) that trigger muscle contractions are derived from animal fat—meat, dairy products, and eggs. The beneficial muscle-relaxant series-1 and series-3 prostaglandins are derived from vegetable and fish sources of fatty acids. These fatty acids, called linoleic acid and alpha-linolenic acid, are found predominantly in raw seeds and nuts, such as flaxseed or pumpkin seed, and certain fish, such as trout, mackerel, and salmon. Thus, how we eat can determine which hormonal pathway we travel—toward muscle tension or muscle relaxation. This is a good example of how our food selection can determine our state of health.

Causes of Endometriosis

Medical research has not pinpointed one specific factor that triggers endometriosis. Instead, a variety of mechanical, hormonal, and immunological triggers may predispose women to developing this complex disease. The most likely theories about the cause of endometriosis are explained in the following paragraphs.

Theory: Menstrual Backup (Retrograde Menstruation). This theory, first proposed in 1921 by a researcher named John A. Simpson, suggests that endometriosis is caused by the backing up of pieces of the uterine lining, or endometrium, during menstruation. That is, instead of exiting through the vagina as part of the menstrual flow, some tissue backs up through the fallopian tubes and into the pelvic cavity. In the pelvis, these pieces of tissue implant onto pelvic organs such as the ovary and bowel. The tissue continues to function as the normal uterine lining would, responding to the cyclical hormonal output from the endocrine glands and bleeding on a monthly basis into the pelvic cavity.

This theory has had support from research done on animals such as monkeys, rabbits, and rats; when endometrial tissue was implanted into their pelvic cavities, the development of endometriosis followed. However, research on women, performed by doing laparoscopies (a surgical technique allowing visualization of the pelvis) during their menstrual periods, has shown that almost all women push blood through their fallopian tubes into the pelvic cavity during menstruation.

Some researchers have suggested that this tendency is more pronounced in women whose uteruses are tipped backward, or retroverted. Other physicians have suggested that menstrual cramps caused by uterine spasm may predispose women toward developing endometriosis. None of these theories has been proven, and not all women develop endometriosis. Obviously, there are other factors that cause the endometrial tissue to implant and cause active disease.

Theory: Spread through Blood Circulation and Lymph Glands. This theory was suggested by a researcher named J. Hilbran to explain why some endometrial implants occasionally are found as far away as a lung or armpit. Rather than invalidating the retro grade menstruation theory, Hilbran's theory simply offers alternate channels through which tissue of the uterine lining can spread to more distant sites. Blood and lymph circulate throughout the body and are natural pathways for the dissemination of endometrial tissue.

This process, known as metastasis, is the same process by which cancer spreads in the body. However, once cancer or endometriosis spreads, the two conditions act entirely differently in their pattern of growth. While cancer consumes and destroys the host organ to which it attaches itself, the endometrial implants use the host as a place to embed themselves and grow.

Theory: Impaired Immune Function. As mentioned earlier, almost all women experience retrograde menstruation, but not all develop endometriosis. Some researchers have postulated that an impaired or altered immune response allows the endometrial implants to grow. Normally, the immune system protects us from disease-causing agents, including viruses, fungi, bacteria, and an array of other foreign invaders such as pollen, dust, pollutants, and chemicals. When the body encounters these agents, the immune system mounts a complex protective response. Our immune system also protects us against aberrant cells that arise within our own body, such as cancer cells, or possibly even aberrant endometrial tissue.

The immune system protects us by destroying these invaders and limiting the damage they can cause in the body, such as inflammation and swelling. The process involves the production of immune cells, including phagocytes, lymphocytes, antibodies, neutrophils, and macrophages. Each of these has a specific role in orchestrating the body's protection against invasion and disease; yet together these various cell types act as a supportive team.

When functioning efficiently, the immune system works beautifully to maintain good health. However, the immune system can become compromised and not perform its protective function effectively when our bodies are exposed to such environmental stresses as the excessive use of alcohol, recreational drugs, cigarettes, poor nutritional habits (with diets that are high in fat, sugar, and caffeinated beverages), and severe emotional upset.

Researchers have theorized that women with endometriosis may have a compromised immune function and are thus unable to halt the spread of endometriosis and limit the damage it causes to the pelvic organs. It is possible that when the immune system is compromised, the endometrial implants are able to spread throughout the pelvic region much more aggressively and are more likely to cause tissue damage, such as inflamemation and scarring. This spread would normally be held in check by healthy immune function. Though research on this issue has not been conclusive, it is possible that compromised immune-system function plays a role in the development and spread of this condition.

Risk Factors That Increase the Likelihood of Endometriosis

Whatever the cause of endometriosis, a number of factors can predispose a woman toward developing this problem. Though endometriosis can occur in women of any type or background during their active reproductive years, it does seem to occur more frequently in high-achieving career women who suffer from significant personal and career stress. Significant stress can disrupt the delicate hormonal balance in women, as well as weaken immune function, which can allow endometrial implants to grow and spread. Childlessness is also a risk factor for endometriosis and, in fact, pregnancy does seem to offer protection against developing the symptoms of this disease. This may be in part because women with multiple pregnancies have fewer menstrual cycles than do childless women, and thus have far less stimulation of the implants by the normal monthly hormonal fluctuations.

Endometriosis occurs primarily in Caucasian women, although many cases are found among women of Asian and African heritage and those of other ethnic and racial backgrounds. A familial predisposition to endometriosis seems to exist, and 8 to 10 percent of patients with endometriosis have mothers or sisters similarly afflicted. Women who suffer from recurrent stress to the immune system, such as chronic infections, may also be more prone to the development and spread of endometriosis. Weakened immune systems may be unable to control the proliferation of the implants as well as the inflammation and scarring that they cause in the pelvic area.

As mentioned earlier, the endometrial implants are stimulated by estrogen. The excessive use of any food that elevates estrogen levels is a risk factor for worsening the spread and symptoms of endometriosis. The liver controls the levels of estrogen circulating through the body. It is responsible for deactivating estrogen chemically so that it can be excreted from the body. If the liver is unable to carry out this task efficiently because of a diet high in alcohol, fat, dairy products, red meat, sugar, and chocolate, estrogen levels can become elevated and worsen endometriosis. To deactivate estrogen, the liver also needs sufficient levels of certain B-complex vitamins, so a vitamin B deficiency can exacerbate the problem. Even obesity can contribute to endometriosis because overweight women tend to produce higher levels of estrogen.

The use of estrogen therapy is contraindicated for women with endometriosis. Such women should not be given estrogen-dominant birth control pills, and estrogen replacement therapy should be used very cautiously during the postmenopausal period. Otherwise, women are at risk of restimulating the implants, which often regress after menopause when estrogen levels decline.

In summary, many of the factors that predispose women to the spread of endometriosis can be modified and even eliminated through changes in lifestyle. This is true even for women whose racial, ethnic, and family background would put them in a higher risk category. The lifestyle modifications that can help eliminate endometriosis are discussed in the self-help section of this book.

Symptoms of Endometriosis

Endometriosis can present with a wide variety of symptoms. The types of symptoms and degree of severity depend on where the implants are located. Interestingly, 30 percent of women with endometriosis experience no symptoms at all and find out only incidentally that they have this problem. Typically this happens if the implants are located away from nerves and other sensitive structures within the pelvis. The other 70 percent of affected women can find endometriosis quite disabling, experiencing severe and recurrent symptoms. The most common symptoms found in women with endometriosis are described in the following paragraphs.

Menstrual Cramps and Pain. Approximately 60 percent of women with endometriosis suffer from progressively worsening menstrual cramps. Menstrual cramp problems caused by endometriosis often begin when women are in their twenties and thirties, although they can affect teenagers, also. Symptoms may occur for as long as two weeks premenstrually and can continue through menstruation. Cramps caused by endometriosis may be extremely painful and may not respond to the usual menstrual cramp medications, such as birth control pills or anti-inflammatory drugs.

The chronic pelvic pain caused by endometriosis may be due not only to stimulation of and bleeding from the implants, but also to the adhesions and pelvic scarring that inflammation in these implants causes over time. Many women with advanced endometriosis are discovered during surgery to have thick scar tissue that can deform or even obliterate the normal structure of the ovaries, ligaments, bowels, and other pelvic structures.

Some women with endometriosis also suffer from pain at ovulation (or mittelschmerz). Mid-month ovulation usually causes no pain in most women. However, in women with endometriosis, hormonal stimulation of the implants can cause a slight bleeding with subsequent irritation of nerve endings in the pelvic cavity. This can lead to pelvic pain lasting about two days.

Dyspareunia. This means pain on sexual intercourse. It can occur when there is endometrial invasion of the uterosacral ligaments or of a pouch located behind the uterus called the cul-de-sac, or pouch of Douglas. Implants growing in this area can push the uterus in a tilted-back position that doctors call retroversion. When the uterus is pulled backward out of its normal position, deep vaginal penetration during intercourse can become very painful. In fact, the pain can be so severe that sexual intercourse becomes too uncomfortable to participate in. Implants in the cul-de-sac can also be responsible for the low back pain that affects some women during menstruation.

Infertility. Endometriosis is a common cause of infertility. Medical studies have estimated that approximately 30 percent of women with endometriosis are unable to conceive. Endometriosis can cause infertility by scarring and obstructing the fallopian tubes so severely that the tubes cannot pick up the egg, or by scarring the ovaries so extensively that ovulation is prevented. In the general population, approximately 10 percent of women are estimated to be infertile. For women who have never been pregnant and still want to conceive and bear a child, this may be one of the more difficult emotional aspects surrounding endometriosis. Accomplishing a successful pregnancy may require long-term medical care, and even this effort does not always succeed.

Medical studies have found, not surprisingly, that the milder the case, the more likely a woman is to become pregnant after treatment of the endometriosis. For example, in one study done using Danazol (a common hormonal therapy for endometriosis, discussed further in Chapter 12), women with milder cases had more than twice the pregnancy rate of those with severe disease. Specifically among women with mild cases of disease, this meant an 83 percent success rate versus a 37 percent success rate within the first year of stopping drug therapy. Still the news is good for women in all stages of the disease, as fertility is a possible and achievable goal for a number of women with endometriosis related infertility.

Abnormal Bleeding. Abnormal bleeding, including premenstrual spotting as well as excessive menstrual flow, occurs in approximately one-third of all women with endometriosis. In some cases of endometriosis, the menstrual cycles may also be irregular. Bleeding abnormalities in women with endometriosis may be due to lack of ovulation.

In anovulatory cycles, progesterone is not secreted. Progesterone has an important effect on the uterine lining during the normal menstrual cycle and helps to limit the amount of blood flow. When progesterone is missing, blood flow can be excessive. When excessive bleeding or spotting happens frequently, iron-deficiency anemia may occur. Women with anemia due to excessive bleeding may find that their energy levels drop and that they lose stamina and endurance, in addition to the other symptoms of endometriosis.

Rectal and Bladder Involvement. When endometrial implants invade the small intestine or colon, unpleasant symptoms may result. Endometrial implants that invade the bowel can cause constipation, painful bowel movements, and rectal bleeding. Since hemorrhoids or even cancer can cause similar symptoms, all symptoms that might be caused by bowel invasion need to be carefully evaluated by a physician. Invasion of the small intestine by endometriosis can cause abdominal swelling, pain, and vomiting.

Occasionally, endometriosis will invade the bladder and cause symptoms similar to urinary tract infections with urinary frequency, pain on urination, urinary retention, and blood in the urine during menstruation.

Endometrial Cysts. These cysts, also called "chocolate cysts;' tend to be deep brown in color, and are filled with old blood and endometrial cells. They can vary greatly in size, ranging from quite small to larger than a grapefruit. They tend to grow fast and even leak blood, which causes much pain. They can also rupture and present with symptoms much like acute appendicitis, a surgical emergency.

In summary, symptoms such as menstrual cramps and pain, pain on sexual intercourse, infertility, abnormal bleeding, bowel and bladder symptoms, and endometrial cysts can occur if you are suffering from endometriosis. How severe the symptoms are depends on the location and extent of the implants. The more mild the symptoms, the easier they are to control with less invasive treatments while more severe symptoms may need more aggressive medical treatment to help relieve your symptoms and control the underlying process of endometriosis.

Happily, I have found that my all-natural treatment program for endometriosis has been very effective in helping to eliminate symptoms of this condition regardless of the degree of your symptoms. I have been thrilled by how much my patients have benefitted from this safe, gentle all-natural approach to treatment.

Symptoms of Endometriosis

- Menstrual pain and cramps
- Pain at ovulation (mittelschmerz)
- Pelvic pain
- Low back pain
- Painful intercourse
- Infertility
- Excessive menstrual bleeding
- Premenstrual spotting
- Menstrual irregularity
- Constipation, painful bowel movements
- Rectal bleeding (especially with menstruation)
- Abdominal pain, swelling, vomiting
- Urinary frequency, pain on urination
- Blood in the urine during menstruation

Risk Factors for Endometriosis

- Childlessness
- High degree of personal and/or career stress
- Caucasian
- Family members with endometriosis
- Immune system stress, such as chronic infections
- Use of estrogen-dominant birth control pills
- Use of estrogen replacement therapy
- Excessive use of alcohol, fat, dairy products, red meat, sugar, chocolate
- Lack of B vitamins
- Obesity

Part II:
Evaluating Your Symptoms

2

The Endometriosis Workbook

An important part of your self-care program is your personal evaluation of your symptoms, possible risk factors and how your lifestyle, including your diet, nutritional status, level of stress and exercise habits may be affecting your symptoms of endometriosis. I have developed this workbook to help you evaluate your symptoms and identify your risk factors that can contribute to endometriosis. This will help you to pinpoint areas of your lifestyle that need to be modified or corrected for better symptom relief.

First, begin to fill out the monthly calendar of endometriosis symptoms, starting today. It is very helpful to make several copies of the calendar. If you recall your symptoms for the past month, chart these symptoms as well. The calendar will enable you to record the types of symptoms you have, as well as evaluate their severity. This will make it easier for you to pick the appropriate treatments for symptom relief. Keep the monthly calendars to check your progress.

After you've started the calendar, turn to the risk factor and lifestyle evaluations that follow the calendar section. They will help you assess specific areas of your life—diet, exercise, stress—to see which of your habit patterns may be contributing to your health problems. I have found that lifestyle habits significantly affect the symptoms of endometriosis.

By filling out the lifestyle evaluation forms, you can easily recognize your weak areas. When you've completed these evaluations, you will be ready to go on to the self-help chapters that follow and begin planning and initiating your personal treatment program. Besides helping you plan your own program, these charts can be useful when you discuss your situation with your physician.

The information contained in these charts about your symptoms, lifestyle habits, and possible risk factors can help your physician assess the severity of your problem as well as determine the need for medical intervention. I have personally found it very helpful when my patients share these charts with me.

Monthly Calendar of Menstrual Symptoms

Grade your symptoms as you experience them each month

○ None   ✔ Mild   ◗ Moderate   ● Severe   Date _____

DAY OF CYCLE	1	2	3	4	5	6	7	8	9	10	11	12	13	14	15	16	17	18	19	20	21	22	23	24	25	26	27	28	29	30	31
Symptom																															
Heavy menstrual bleeding																															
Spotting																															
Spasmodic menstrual cramps/pain																															
Low back pain																															
Premenstrual pain up to two weeks prior																															
Pain in inner thighs																															
Abdominal tenderness																															
Nausea and vomiting																															
Diarrhea																															
Constipation																															
Bloating																															
Hot and Cold																															
Faintness, dizziness																															
Fatigue																															
Headaches																															
Sleeplessness																															
Pain in midcycle (mittleschmerz)																															
Pain during or after intercourse																															
Rectal bleeding																															
Urinary frequency																															
Blood in urine																															

Risk Factors for Endometriosis

You are at higher risk of developing endometriosis and suffering from symptoms caused by either of these problems if you have any of the following risk factors. Be sure to follow the nutritional, exercise, and stress management guidelines in the self-help section of this book if any of the related risk factors apply to you. Check each risk factor that applies to you.

Risk Factors

Career or working woman _____

High-stress life, combining work and child care _____

Age twenties through forties _____

Multiple pregnancies _____

Tendency toward ovarian cysts that bleed _____

Mothers or sisters with a history of endometriosis _____

High levels of estrogen as determined by your physician, or use of estrogen-containing medication _____

High levels of prostaglandin hormones as determined by your physician _____

Repeated laparoscopies significant life stress _____

Emotional distress that hampers well-being, anxiety, depression _____

Concurrent immune stress, recurrent or chronic infections, allergies _____

High dietary intake of meat, saturated fat, dairy products, alcohol, sugar, caffeine, salt, or chocolate _____

Lack of B vitamins _____

Lack of exercise _____

Eating Habits and Endometriosis

All the foods in the shaded area of the following list are high-stress foods that can worsen the symptoms of both problems. If you eat many of these foods, or if you eat any of these foods frequently, your nutritional habits may be contributing significantly to your symptoms. Read the chapters on dietary principles and meal plans and recipes for further guidance on food selection.

All the foods from avocado to fish are high-nutrient, low-stress foods that may help to relieve or prevent and endometriosis symptoms. Include these foods frequently in your diet. If you are already eating many of these foods and few of the high-stress foods, chances are your nutritional habits are good, and food selection may not be a significant factor in worsening your or endometriosis. You may want to look carefully at the stress management and exercise chapters. The activities contained in these chapters may be very helpful in relieving your symptoms.

Eating Habits Checklist

Check the number of times you eat the following foods.

Foods That Increase Symptoms

Foods	Never	1x a Month	1x a Week	>1x a Week
Coffee				
Cow's milk				
Cow's cheese				
Butter				
Chocolate				
Sugar				
Alcohol				
Wheat bread				
Wheat noodles				
Wheat-based flour				
Pastries				
Added salt				
Bouillon				
Commercial salad dressing				
Catsup				
Black tea				
Soft drinks				
Hot dogs				
Ham				
Bacon				
Beef				
Lamb				
Pork				

Foods That Decrease Symptoms

Foods	Never	1x a Month	1x a Week	>1x a Week
Avocado				
Green Beans				
Beets				
Broccoli				
Brussels sprouts				
Cabbage				
Carrots				
Celery				
Collard greens				
Cucumbers				
Eggplant				
Garlic				
Horseradish				
Kale				
Legumes				
Lettuce				
Mustard greens				
Okra				
Onions				
Parsnips				
Peas				
Potatoes				
Radishes				
Rutabagas				
Spinach				
Squash				
Sweet potatoes				
Tomatoes				
Turnips				
Turnip greens				
Yams				
Brown rice				
Millet				
Barley				
Oatmeal				
Buckwheat				
Rye				
Raw flaxseeds				
Corn				

Raw pumpkin seeds				
Raw sesame seeds				
Raw sunflower seeds				
Raw almonds				
Raw filberts				
Raw pecans				
Raw walnuts				
Apples				
Bananas				
Berries				
Pears				
Seasonal fruits				
Corn oil				
Flax oil				
Olive oil				
Sesame oil				
Safflower oil				
Eggs				
Poultry				
Fish				

Exercise Habits and Endometriosis

Exercise helps prevent the pain and cramps related to endometriosis by relaxing muscles and promoting better blood circulation and oxygenation to the pelvic area. Exercise can also help reduce stress and relieve anxiety and upset. If your total number of exercise periods per week is less than three, you will probably be prone to pain and cramp symptoms. See the chapters on the various kinds of exercise that can help relieve and prevent symptoms.

If you are exercising more than three times a week, keep doing your exercises; they are probably making your symptoms less severe. You may want to add specific corrective exercises to your present regime, choosing them to fit your individual symptoms.

You will find many options available in the chapters on exercise, stretches, and acupressure massage.

Exercise Checklist

Check the frequency with which you do any of the following:

Exercise	Never	1x a Month	1x a Week	>1x a Week
Walking				
Running				
Dancing				
Swimming				
Bicycling				
Tennis				
Stretching				

Stress and Endometriosis

Checking many items in the first third of the following scale indicates major life stress and a possible vulnerability to serious illness. In other words, the more items checked in the first third, the higher your stress quotient. Do everything possible to manage your stress in a healthy way. Eat the foods that provide a high-nutrient/low stress diet, exercise on a regular basis, and learn the methods for managing stress given in the chapters on stress reduction and deep breathing.

If you have checked fewer items, you are probably at low risk of illness caused by stress. But because stresses too small to figure in this evaluation may also play a part in worsening your endometriosis symptoms, you would still benefit from practicing the methods outlined in the chapter on stress reduction. Stress management is very important in helping you gain control over your level of muscle tension.

Major Stress Evaluation

Check each stressful event that applies to you.

Life Events

_____ Death of spouse or close family member

_____ Divorce from spouse

_____ Death of a close friend

_____ Legal separation from spouse

_____ Loss of job

_____ Radical loss of financial security

_____ Major personal injury or illness (gynecologic or other cause)

_____ Future surgery for gynecologic or other illness

_____ Beginning a new marriage

_____ Foreclosure of mortgage or loan

_____ Lawsuit lodged against you

_____ Marriage reconciliation

_____ Change in health of a family member

_____ Major trouble with boss or co-workers

_____ Increase in responsibility—job or home

_____ Learning you are pregnant

_____ Difficulties with your sexual abilities

_____ Gaining a new family member

_____ Change to a different job

_____ Increase in number of marital arguments

_____ New loan or mortgage of more than $100,000

_____ Son or daughter leaving home

_____ Major disagreement with in-laws or friends

_____ Recognition for outstanding achievements

_____ Spouse begins or stops work

_____ Begin or end education

_____ Undergo a change in living conditions

_____ Revise or alter your personal habits

_____ Change in work hours or conditions

_____ Change of residence

_____ Change your school or major in school

_____ Alterations in your recreational activities

_____ Change in church or club activities

_____ Change in social activities

_____ Change in sleeping habits

_____ Change in number of family get-togethers

_____ Diet or eating habits are changed

_____ You go on vacation

_____ The year-end holidays occur

_____ You commit a minor violation of the law

Major life stress can have a significant impact on the symptoms of endometriosis as well as other health problems. It is helpful to assess your level of stress to see how it may be affecting your health. One popular tool is the Holmes and Rahe Social Readjustment Rating Scale, which gives you a stress "score." The scale above is adapted for women and simply identifies major life events that cause stress.

Daily Stress Evaluation

This evaluation is a very important one for women with endometriosis. Not all stresses have a major impact in our lives, as do death, divorce, or personal injury. Most of us are exposed to a multitude of small life stresses on a daily basis. The effects of these stresses are cumulative and can be a major factor in worsening endometriosis-related muscle tension and pain in the pelvic area. After completing the checklist, read over the day-to-day stress areas that you find difficult to handle. Becoming aware of them is the first step toward lessening their effects on your life. Methods for reducing them and helping your body to deal with them are given in Chapter 7.

Check each item that seems to apply to you.

Work

____ **Too much responsibility.** You feel you have to push too hard to do your work. There are too many demands made of you. You feel very pressured by all of this responsibility. You worry about getting all your work done and doing it well.

____ **Time urgency.** You worry about getting your work done on time. You always feel rushed. It feels like there are not enough hours in the day to complete your work.

____ **Job instability.** You are concerned about losing your job. There are layoffs at your company. There is much insecurity and concern among your fellow employees about their job security.

____ **Job performance.** You don't feel that you are working up to your maximum capability due to outside pressures or stress. You are unhappy with your job performance and concerned about job security as a result.

____ **Difficulty getting along with co-workers and boss.** Your boss is too picky and critical. Your boss demands too much. You must work closely with co-workers who are difficult to get along with.

____ **Understimulation.** Work is boring. The lack of stimulation makes you tired. You wish you were some-where else.

____ **Uncomfortable physical plant.** Lights are too bright or too dim; noises are too loud. You're exposed to noxious fumes or chemicals. There is too much activity going on around you, making it difficult to concentrate.

Spouse or Significant Other

____ **Hostile communication.** There is too much negative emotion and drama. You are always upset and angry. There is not enough peace and quiet.

____ **Not enough communication.** There is not enough discussion of feelings or issues. You both tend to hold in your feelings. You feel that an emotional bond is lacking between you.

____ **Discrepancy in communication.** One person talks about feelings too much, the other person too little.

____ **Affection.** You do not feel you receive enough affection. There is not enough holding, touching, and loving in your relationship. Or, you are made uncomfortable by your partner's demands.

____ **Sexuality.** There is not enough sexual intimacy. You feel deprived by your partner. Or, your partner demands sexual relations too often. You feel pressured.

____ **Children.** They make too much noise. They make too many demands on your time. They are hard to discipline.

____ **Organization.** Home is poorly organized. It always seems messy; chores are half-finished.

____ **Time.** There is too much to do in the home and never enough time to get it all done.

____ **Responsibility.** You need more help. There are too many demands on your time and energy.

Your Emotional State

____ **Too much anxiety.** You worry too much about every little thing. You constantly worry about what can go wrong in your life.

____ **Victimization.** Everyone is taking advantage of you or wants to hurt you.

____ **Poor self-image.** You don't like yourself enough. You are always finding fault with yourself.

____ **Too critical.** You are always finding fault with others. You always look at what is wrong with other people rather than seeing their virtues.

____ **Inability to relax.** You are always wound up. It is difficult for you to relax. You are tense and restless.

____ **Not enough self-renewal.** You don't play enough or take enough time off to relax and have fun. Life isn't fun and enjoyable as a result.

____ **Feeling of depression.** You feel blue, isolated, and tearful. You feel a sense of self-blame and hopelessness. Fatigue and low energy are problems.

____ **Too angry.** Small life issues seem to upset you unduly. You find yourself becoming angry and irritable with your husband, children, or clients.

How Stress Affects Your Body

The following checklist should help you become aware of where stress localizes in your body. Each woman accumulates stress in a different way, tensing and contracting different sets of muscles in a pattern unique to her. Storing tension in the low back and pelvic area can worsen cramps, while storing it in the neck can cause headaches. This accumulation also increases your level of fatigue and lowers your energy and vitality.

Check the places where tension most commonly localizes in your body.

____   Low back
____   Pelvic area
____   Stomach muscles
____   Thighs and calves
____   Chest
____   Shoulders Arms
____   Neck and throat
____   Headache
____   Grinding teeth
____   Eyestrain

It is important to be aware of where you store tension. When you feel tension building up in these areas, begin deep breathing (Chapter 8) or use one of the stress-reduction techniques given in Chapter 7. Often, these techniques will help release muscle tension rapidly.

3

Medical Testing For Endometriosis

If you suspect that you have endometriosis, it is very important to have a thorough diagnostic evaluation done to confirm that you actually have this condition and to pinpoint its extent and severity. This will help to differentiate this condition from other causes of pelvic and abdominal pain, bleeding and even infertility. It will also assist in helping you and your caregiver in deciding what will be the most effective treatments for this condition to provide relief for your symptoms or remove any block to becoming pregnant if infertility has been an issue.

There are five possible steps that your physician or caregiver may need to take in order to accurately diagnose this condition. This includes taking a medical history, doing a pelvic exam, and a laparoscopy or surgical evaluation of the problem. There are also other noninvasive diagnostic techniques, depending on the extent and location of your endometriosis lesions, as well as blood or saliva hormone testing.

I am going to describe the process of diagnosing endometriosis in some detail so that you can know what to expect once you start this process. Let's look now at each of these steps.

Medical History

Your doctor will always begin the process of evaluating your cause of menstrual pain or other possible symptoms of endometriosis by taking a careful medical history. This should include questions about your menstrual cycle, how many days your period lasts and how often it occurs. Your caregiver should find out how heavy is your bleeding including how often you change your pad or tampons and if you have any spotting in between your periods.

It is also essential to find out about the location and severity of any pain or cramping and when it occurs in relationship to your period as well as any pain at mid-cycle, the time of ovulation. There can also be pain on sexual intercourse with deep penetration. Since endometriosis lesions can implant in different organ system, your caregiver should also ask you about any bowel, digestive or bladder symptoms as well as your fertility and any pregnancies.

Risk factors such as other family members with endometriosis, your use of hormones, your dietary and nutritional status and your level of personal, work and family stress should also be evaluated. Unfortunately, these essential lifestyle factors are more likely to be looked at and evaluated by an alternative health practitioner rather than a conventional medical doctor.

Pelvic Exam

Next, your doctor should do a pelvic exam can help to determine the shape and size of your uterus, cervix and ovaries and help to diagnose the presence of endometriosis cysts and implants. A pelvic exam can also help to detect and rule out other obvious causes of bleeding and pain such as cervical erosion, polyps, or fibroid tumors.

If your pelvic exam is normal, the uterus, cervix, ovaries and fallopian tubes should be normal in size and location. Your uterus can be moved slightly when doing the exam without causing any pain and no other pelvic pain or tenderness is present. No cysts or hardening of the tissue will be felt and no abnormal tissue is felt in the cul-de-sac (this is the area between the uterus and rectum) or in the ligaments that hold the uterus in place.

If you do have endometriosis, there are a number of physical signs that can be noted during a pelvic exam by an experienced gynecologist. Sometimes, the uterus is fixed and not freely mobile; it can also be retroverted, or tilted backward. The endometriosis implants may cause pain, tenderness and cramping, depending on their location within the pelvic cavity.

Your ovaries may be enlarged because of the presence of endometrial or chocolate cysts. Sometimes these cysts may be large and easy to feel. Your ovaries may also be painful when touched or not freely movable if you have scar tissue or adhesions. Scar tissue around the fallopian tubes and ovaries can block the tubes or interfere with their ability to pick up the egg and be a cause of infertility.

Endometrial implants located in the uterosacral ligaments will feel nodular and shotty (hard and round, like a shot pellet) on examination. These are ligaments on each side of the uterus that extend from the cervix to the sacrum and help to stabilize the uterus. Tenderness in these ligaments is particularly noted at the time of menstruation.

Your caregiver should do a rectal exam to evaluate if there are endometriosis implants present in the cul-de-sac (the area between the uterus and rectum). You may have nodularity, pain and tenderness when your caregiver does an exam of this area. Nodularity in this area is typical of endometriosis and occurs when the implants and scar tissue fuse the rectum to the back of the vagina.

A Pap smear should be done at this time, if you have not had one recently as well as a general physical exam to evaluate the location or spread of the endometriosis implants as well as your general level of health and well-being.

Laparoscopy and Other Evaluation Techniques

Laparoscopy. For a definitive diagnosis of endometriosis, a surgical procedure called a laparoscopy is usually necessary. The laparoscope is a visualization device shaped like a thin tube. This device allows your gynecologist to actually look at all of your reproductive organs within the pelvic cavity and see if any obvious endometriosis implants or scar tissue is present.

During the procedure, the laparoscopic device is inserted through a small abdominal incision. Gas is introduced into the abdomen to move the organs apart for better visualization of any disease process. This also allows the physician to see the ovaries and fallopian tubes. Laparoscopy enables the physician to see any lesions that have the typical appearance of endometriosis implants; puckered "powder burn" lesions, red lesions, and blueberry colored spots may commonly be seen, as well as white scar tissue, or adhesions, and chocolate ovarian cysts.

Laparoscopy can also be used to determine if fertilization is impaired by the implants. By infusing a bluish colored dye through the fallopian tubes, the degree of openness (or patency) of the tubes can be evaluated. This is important if you have been trying to become pregnant and if possible infertility caused by endometriosis is an issue.

Surgical treatment can usually be initiated at the time of laparoscopy. Adhesions and implants can be dissolved with a laser or by electro-cauterization. However, there are women with endometriosis for whom laparoscopy is not advisable. These include patients with extensive endometriosis, massive scarring, or implants that have invaded deep into the ovaries, urinary tract, or bowels. These patients will often require more extensive surgery.

Culdoscopy. A similar technique called culdoscopy may also be performed. Culdoscopy was a more common diagnostic tool before the introduction of laparoscopy, which has superseded it in recent years. Unlike laparoscopy, culdoscopy must be done through an incision in the vaginal wall. A periscope-like instrument is introduced through this incision and allows a view of the uterus, ovaries, and fallopian tubes. A woman must be placed in an awkward position for the exam, which should be done under a local anesthetic. The intestines tend to fall forward with this exam, so the area behind the uterus is better visualized. However, this technique involves a somewhat higher risk of infection than laparoscopy, and it allows a more limited range of procedures to be performed.

Noninvasive Techniques

Ultrasound. Other imaging techniques may give additional clues to the locations of the endometrial implants. Your physician may also recommend an imaging technique called an ultrasound. Unlike laparoscopy, ultrasound is a noninvasive technique that allows visualization of pelvic structures such as the uterus and ovaries by bouncing high-frequency sound waves off these solid masses. The waves bounce back in patterns that appear as pictures on a screen.

Ultrasound can visualize the size and shape of any pelvic masses like ovarian cysts and large implants due to endometriosis This technique is particularly helpful in diagnosing chocolate ovarian cysts. Ultrasound can also be used to assess the thickness of the uterine lining in the diagnosis of hyperplasia. Once the cause of the bleeding is accurately pinpointed, the appropriate treatment can be prescribed.

Magnetic Resonance Imaging (MRI). MRI is a technique that uses both a magnetic field and radio waves to create detailed images of the organs and tissues of your body. MRI devices are actually large tube-shaped magnets that you lie inside of while the magnetic field temporarily aligns the water molecules of your body. At the same time, the radio waves cause these aligned particles to produce signals to create three-dimensional images of your organs and tissues that may be viewed from many different angles.

While endometriosis is definitively diagnosed by laparoscopy, sometimes an MRI is also done to help determine the extent of the endometriosis. It is especially useful in evaluating the presence of deep infiltrating lesions. An MRI is likely to be done when laparoscopic visualization is limited by scar tissue or adhesions. It is also very helpful in diagnosing endometrial or chocolate cysts and invasion of the colon wall by endometriosis implants.

Cystoscopy. In women with symptoms such as urinary frequency, blood in the urine at menstruation, and bladder pain, all of which suggest endometrial invasion of the bladder wall, specific evaluation techniques of the genitourinary tract may be necessary. Imaging of the genitourinary tract may be done with cystoscopy. In cystoscopy, a visualizing scope is inserted through the urethra into the bladder. Blockage or invasion of the urethra and bladder can be seen with this device.

Intravenous Pyelogram. Your physician may also order an intravenous pyelogram (IVP) to evaluate if endometriosis implants have invaded your kidneys. An IVP that targets the kidneys requires injecting dye into a vein. When the dye travels to the kidneys, X-rays are then taken. This technique reveals an endometrial invasion of the kidneys as a telltale indentation. However, this technique does not specifically allow a diagnosis of endometriosis to be made, because other conditions, such as cancer, can also invade kidney tissue. In this case, further evaluation may be necessary for a definitive diagnosis.

Barium enema. An X-ray called a barium enema may help to better visualize endometrial growths in the intestines, especially the colon. This procedure is usually done if your physician suspects severe endometriosis in the bowels. A chalky, opaque liquid is passed through the colon and allows any growths or deformities to be seen by X-rays. This procedure can be helpful in accurately diagnosing bowel wall invasion by endometriosis implants and even helping to ensure proper surgical planning, if more extensive surgery is going to be done to treat this condition.

Blood and Saliva Testing

Your doctor may also want to order laboratory testing to check your hormone levels, particularly your estrogen and progesterone levels since the implants are stimulated by high estrogen levels and their growth is limited by progesterone.

Until the 1990's, the method for checking women's hormone levels had severe limitations. A single blood sample was taken and analyzed, though the results of this one-time check were unhelpful, given the ebb and flow of your hormone levels throughout the month. In addition, the stress of having blood drawn was enough to throw off a woman's hormone levels and skew the results.

Fortunately, female hormone testing done through saliva samples are also now commonly available. Saliva testing is not only non-invasive (no needle sticks!), but it is also highly accurate. These tests can help to evaluate your hormonal status and assist in the design of an individualized treatment program for your endometriosis symptoms that can deliver the maximum benefits with minimum risk of side effects.

Best of all, saliva hormone testing is accessible. Even physicians who still don't routinely order saliva hormone testing will usually do so if a patient requests it. You can even order a limited saliva hormone test kit on your own directly from a laboratory, without a doctor's prescription.

Like blood, saliva closely mirrors hormone levels in your body's tissues. However, saliva is a particularly accurate indicator of free (unbound) hormone levels. This is the key, as only free hormones are active, meaning that they can affect the hormone-sensitive tissues in your breasts, brain, heart, and uterus. Saliva testing therefore provides a superior measure of the levels of hormones that actually affect vital body systems, mood, tissue levels of sodium and fluid, and many other important functions.

Additionally, blood testing only provides a one-time "snapshot" of hormone levels, whereas saliva testing provides a dynamic picture of hormonal ebb and flow over an entire menstrual cycle. In fact, saliva samples are collected during the month, all at the same time of day, and then sent to a laboratory. The lab measures and charts your progesterone and estradiol (your most prevalent and potent form of estrogen) levels. These results are compared to normal patterns. Finally, saliva testing is easy, stress-free and non-invasive. You can collect your own saliva samples, which means you don't have to go to your doctor's office or a lab. Plus, there's no need to draw blood.

If you think saliva hormone testing is right for you, consider consulting your physician. Having your doctor order the test has two advantages: The profile is more extensive, and your insurance may cover the cost. A number of laboratories perform the test. If your doctor doesn't order the test, or you simply want insight to help you develop your own self-care regimen, you can order a test kit from laboratories through the Internet. A complete blood count may also be ordered by your doctor to check for anemia, as well as a chemistry panel to establish your general health.

Part III:
Finding the Solution

4

Dietary Principles for Relief of Endometriosis

I cannot emphasize too strongly the importance of good dietary habits for women beginning an endometriosis treatment program. After years of working with thousands of women patients suffering from this condition, I have found that no therapy can be fully effective without including beneficial dietary changes as part of the treatment plan.

My endometriosis relief diet can help to bring estrogen back into balance by reducing estrogen production by the ovaries and adrenal glands as well as interfering with estrogen's ability to bind to tissue receptors. The proper diet can also support the breakdown and detoxification of estrogen by the liver and promote its elimination from the body through the intestinal tract.

I developed the dietary plan discussed in this chapter as a result of working with thousands of patients who came to me for help in resolving their endometriosis symptoms and have found it to be very successful. This is the diet in a nutshell:

Eat a vegetarian emphasis diet with plenty of fresh vegetables, fruits, whole grains, legumes, raw seeds and nuts, and healthy monounsaturated oils like olive oil and almond oil. However, if you feel your best on a meat-based, higher protein intake diet, red meat should be avoided since it contains inflammation causing saturated fat. Animal sources of protein should include free-range poultry, eggs and omega-3 fatty acid rich fish like salmon, trout and halibut. Omega-3 fatty acids actually help to reduce inflammation. Foods should be eaten raw or lightly steamed with a minimum of rich sauces and dressings.

Some women feel their best on a high complex carbohydrate, whole grain based diet while other women need a much higher, meat protein intake. Either type of diet is fine, as long as you include the foods that are therapeutic for this condition and will help to bring your hormones back into balance, while eliminating the "bad" offending foods that will worsen your symptoms. In the recipe and meal planning section, I include both complex carbohydrate and protein-based dishes.

Include foods, such as buckwheat, whole citrus fruit pulp (not just the juice), and ground flax meal in shakes and cereals. If you tolerate and enjoy soy foods, they can be helpful, too, in balancing excess estrogen levels within the body. These foods help to reduce estrogen production and prevent this hormone from binding to tissue receptors. Flaxseed also helps to promote healthy progesterone production.

Avoid fried and fatty foods like potato chips, pizza, ice cream and cheese. In addition, avoid caffeine, alcohol, chocolate, sugar, soft drinks, fruit juices and salt. All of these foods hamper the process of detoxification by the liver. Healthy detoxification is necessary to metabolize estrogens to safer and less potent forms.

Eat a low-fat, high-fiber diet to help your intestines eliminate excess estrogen so it is not reabsorbed back into your body. Include plenty of fresh fruits, vegetables, ground flaxseed, whole grains, and legumes (beans and peas).

Reduce or eliminate red meats; they not only elevate estrogen levels but also contain the type of fats that cause menstrual cramps and worsen the inflammation of endometriosis. Instead, eat fish such as salmon, mackerel, sardines, trout and tuna, which are high in beneficial omega-3 fatty acids that reduce the pain of menstrual cramps and endometriosis. Free-range chicken or turkey are also good dietary options. In addition, instead of hamburgers and hot dogs, buy vegetarian-based substitutes.

Avoid wheat and dairy products since they worsen inflammation and have a negative effect on reproductive health similar to that of red meat. Instead of wheat use gluten-free bread, bagels, muffins, crackers and pastries made from rice, quinoa, millet, buckwheat or other gluten-free flours. Use soy, rice, almond, coconut, flaxseed, hemp and sunflower seed dairy substitutes, including nondairy milk, cream cheese, sour cream, frozen desserts and yogurt.

Many women have reported significant relief of their symptoms, such as a noticeable decrease in heavy bleeding as well as their pain and discomfort level within one or two menstrual cycles after starting my program.

Foods That Help Treat or Prevent Endometriosis

Let's look at the foods summarized above in more detail. The following foods will provide the range of nutrients that you need to help balance your hormones, reduce your estrogen level, decrease cramping and inflammation, and generally improve your physical and mental well-being. Even though endometriosis symptoms are worse during the second half of the menstrual cycle, these healthful foods should form the mainstay of your diet throughout the entire month. A poorly chosen high-stress diet during your symptom-free time will increase the severity of your symptoms when menstruation starts.

Whole Grains. I strongly recommend the use of certain whole grains such as brown rice, millet, buckwheat, gluten-free oats, wild rice and amaranth. However, wheat and rye need to be avoided because they contain an inflammatory protein called gluten. (I discuss this more in the next section.)

Whole grains are excellent sources of the vitamin B-complex and vitamin E, both of which are important for healthy hormonal balance and lowering excessive estrogen levels through their beneficial effect on both the liver and ovaries. This can help to control the stimulatory effect excessive estrogen has on endometriosis implants.

Whole grains provide other benefits for endometriosis sufferers. The fiber in whole grains binds to estrogen and helps remove it from the body through bowel elimination. This benefit of whole grain fiber was reported in the *New England Journal of Medicine*. In this study, it was found that vegetarian women who eat a high-fiber, low-fat diet have lower blood estrogen levels than omnivorous women with low-fiber diets. Fiber can also help decrease the congestive symptoms of cramps since it produces bulkier stools with a higher water content. This helps to eliminate excessive fluid from the body.

Fiber may also be helpful in reducing the digestive symptoms that occur with endometriosis, since it has a normalizing effect on the bowel movements. Besides removing excessive estrogen, whole grains help to bind dietary fat and cholesterol and eliminate them from the body. Oat and rice bran are very good for this purpose. Because cancers of the breast, uterus, ovaries, and colon are linked to a diet high in animal fats, the use of a low-fat whole grain diet may have a protective effect.

Buckwheat is also beneficial because it contains bioflavonoids that help to lower the production of excess estrogen in the body. Bioflavonoids, which are also found in citrus fruit pulp and rind, help to regulate estrogen levels within the body. I discuss the mechanism of how this process works in the section on fruit as well as the chapter on nutritional supplements if you would like to understand this in more detail.

In addition, whole grains are excellent sources of protein, especially when combined with beans and peas. I strongly recommend vegetable sources of protein since such proteins are easily digestible. Grains are also especially high in magnesium, which helps reduce the neuromuscular tension and thereby decreases menstrual cramps. They are fairly high in calcium, which relaxes muscle contraction. They are excellent sources of potassium. Potassium has a diuretic effect on the body tissues and helps reduce bloating.

Legumes. The best legumes to eat for relief of endometriosis symptoms are soybeans. This includes soy products like tofu, tempeh, boiled soybeans, soy pasta, soy yogurt and soy cheese.

The use of soybeans in the diet helps to regulate and lower estrogen levels in the body. This is because soy is a rich source of natural plant estrogens, called isoflavones. The isoflavones found in soybeans have a chemical structure similar to estrogen, yet are much weaker in potency than the estrogen made by our bodies. (Isoflavones have only 1 /50,000 the potency of synthetic estrogen.) Utilized in the diet, isoflavones actually compete with our body's own estrogen for binding to the estrogen receptors of our cells. Thus the weaker isoflavones can actually replace our own estrogen when binding to the uterus, breasts, and other estrogen-sensitive tissue. Isoflavones can also help lower estrogen levels in the body by actually interfering with estrogen production. Total isoflavone intake should equal 50 to 100 mg per day.

The use of soy foods or the use of isoflavones in a purified form has been found to help reduce bleeding problems in premenopausal women who are not ovulating. As women move into menopause, which occurs when estrogen levels finally drop significantly, isoflavones provide weak estrogen support to the bones, heart, vagina and other tissues of the body.

Unfortunately, many women are either allergic to soy or do not digest soy foods well. They find that when eating soy products, they develop uncomfortable symptoms of indigestion. If this is the case with you, you should avoid soy products entirely and, instead, choose other protein options.

Beans and peas are excellent sources of calcium, magnesium and potassium, which help to reduce the symptoms of pain and cramping seen commonly with endometriosis. I highly recommend their dietary use for endometriosis relief.

Particularly good choices include black beans, pinto beans, kidney beans, chickpeas, lentils, lima beans and soybeans (if you tolerate them well). These foods are also high in iron and tend to be good sources of copper and zinc. Women with endometriosis who suffer from heavy bleeding are often deficient in these minerals, particularly iron. Legumes are also very high in vitamin B-complex and vitamin B6. These are necessary nutrients for healthy liver function, reducing excess estrogen levels, and prevention of cramps and menstrual fatigue. They are also excellent sources of protein and can be used as substitutes for meat at many meals. Legumes provide all the essential amino acids when eaten with grains. Good examples of grain and legume combinations include meals such as beans and rice, or cooked whole grain quinoa and split pea soup.

Like grains, legumes are a good source of fiber and can help normalize bowel function and lower cholesterol. They digest slowly and can help to regulate the blood sugar level, a trait they share with whole grains. As a result, they are an excellent food for women with diabetes or blood sugar imbalances. Some women find that gas is a problem when they eat beans. You can minimize gas by using digestive enzymes, adding powdered ginger to beans as they are cooking, and of course, eating beans in small quantities.

Vegetables. These are outstanding foods for relief of endometriosis symptoms of all types. Many vegetables are high in calcium, magnesium, and potassium, which help to relieve and prevent the spasmodic symptoms of cramps. Besides helping relax tense, irritable muscles, these minerals help calm and relax the emotions, too. Both calcium and magnesium act as natural tranquilizers, a real benefit for women suffering from menstrual pain, discomfort, and irritability. The potassium content of vegetables helps to relieve the symptoms of menstrual congestion by reducing fluid retention and bloating. Some of the best sources for these minerals include Swiss chard, spinach, broccoli, beet greens, mustard greens, sweet potatoes, kale, potatoes, green peas, and green beans. These vegetables are also high in iron, which may help reduce bleeding and cramps.

Many vegetables are high in vitamin C, which helps decrease capillary fragility and facilitate the flow of essential nutrients into the tight muscles as well as the flow of waste products out. When capillaries are strengthened, there is a reduction in the heavy menstrual bleeding commonly seen with endometriosis.

Vitamin C is an important anti-stress vitamin because it is needed for healthy adrenal hormonal production (the adrenals are important glands that help the body deal with stress). It is also important for immune function and wound healing. As a result, vitamin C may help limit scarring and inflammation caused in the pelvis by the endometrial implants. Its anti-infectious properties may reduce bladder and vaginal infections. Vegetables high in vitamin C include Brussels sprouts, broccoli, cauliflower, kale, peppers, parsley, peas, tomatoes and potatoes.

Fruits. Like many vegetables, fruits are an excellent source of vitamin C. This nutrient prevents capillary fragility and reduces heavy menstrual flow. By strengthening blood vessels, it promotes good blood circulation into the tense pelvic muscles. Almost all fruits contain some vitamin C, with the best sources being berries, oranges, grapefruits, and melons. The pulp and rind of citrus fruits are also good sources of bioflavonoids, which also help to fortify capillaries and decrease excessive menstrual bleeding.

Bioflavonoids, interestingly enough, are both weakly estrogenic and anti-estrogenic. Although bioflavonoids are weakly estrogenic themselves, they interfere with the production of estrogen by competing with estrogen precursors for binding sites on the enzymes that normally allow the male hormones testosterone and androstenedione to be converted into estrogen. (This occurs both in the ovary and the fatty tissues of the body. Thus, bioflavonoids help to normalize the body's estrogen levels. They help elevate estrogen levels when they are too low, as seen in menopausal women, and help bring down excessive estrogen levels when they are too high, as can occur in women with endometriosis.

This normalizing effect of the bioflavonoids has been shown in a variety of interesting studies. While bioflavonoids help reduce the hot flashes and night sweats of menopause, they also act to control heavy menstrual bleeding in conditions such as premenopause. Unlike prescription estrogen, the potency of the flavonoids is so weak that they rarely cause side effects.

Certain fruits are also excellent sources of calcium and magnesium; you can eat them often in small amounts to help supply your mineral needs and reduce menstrual pain and cramping. These include dried figs, raisins, blackberries, bananas, and oranges. Figs, raisins, and bananas are also exceptional sources of potassium, so should be eaten by women with fatigue and bloating. All fruits are an excellent source of potassium. Eat fruits whole to take advantage of their high fiber content. Their fiber content helps prevent constipation and the other digestive irregularities frequently seen with menstrual pain and cramps.

Fresh and dried fruits are excellent snack and dessert substitutes for cookies, candies, cakes and other foods high in refined sugar. Though fruit is high in sugar, its high fiber content slows down absorption of the sugar into the blood circulation and helps stabilize the blood sugar level. I recommend, however, using fruit juices only in small quantities. Fruit juice does not contain the bulk or fiber of the whole fruit. As a result, it acts more like table sugar and can dramatically destabilize your blood sugar level when used in excess. In this case, less is better. If you want fruit juice on a more frequent basis, mix it half-and-half with water.

Seeds and Nuts. Raw seeds and nuts are excellent sources of the two essential fatty acids, linoleic acid and alpha-linolenic acid. These acids provide the raw materials your body needs to produce the muscle-relaxant prostaglandin hormones. Adequate levels of essential fatty acids in your diet are very important in treating and preventing endometriosis-related muscle cramps and inflammation. The best sources of both fatty acids are raw flax and pumpkin seeds. Sesame and sunflower seeds are excellent sources of linoleic acid alone.

Seeds and nuts are also excellent sources of the B-complex vitamins and vitamin E, important anti-stress factors for women with cramps; these nutrients also help to regulate hormonal balance. Seeds and nuts are also very high in other essential nutrients that women need, such as magnesium, calcium and potassium. Particularly good to eat are sesame seeds, sunflower seeds, pistachios, pecans and almonds. Because they are very high in calories, seeds and nuts should be eaten in small amounts.

The oils in seeds and nuts are very perishable, so avoid exposure to light, heat and oxygen. Seeds and nuts should be eaten raw and unsalted to get the benefit of their essential fatty acids (which are good for your skin and hair) as well as to avoid the negative effects of too much salt. Shell them yourself, when possible. If you buy them already shelled, refrigerate them so their oils don't become rancid. They are a wonderful garnish on salads, vegetable dishes, and casseroles. They can also be eaten as a main source of protein in snacks and light meals.

Poultry and Fish. I generally recommend eating meat in moderation. Particularly good sources of protein are omega-3 fatty acid containing fish like salmon, tuna, trout, halibut and mackerel. Fish should be eaten no more than once or twice a week due to the high mercury content in most fish. Also good are free-range poultry and eggs. If you want to eat red meat, I recommend choosing organic lean red meat, if grass fed, and game meat. Fatty cuts of beef, pork, and lamb contain saturated fats that produce the muscle-contracting F2 Alpha prostaglandins. These hormones trigger muscle contraction and constriction in blood vessels, as well as inflammation, thereby worsening endometriosis-related cramps and the spread of endometrial implants.

Fish, unlike other meat, contains omega-3 fatty acids that help to relax muscles through the beneficial prostaglandin pathway—specifically, the series-3 prostaglandins. Fish are also excellent sources of minerals, especially iodine and potassium. Particularly good types of fish for women with menstrual cramps are salmon, tuna, halibut, mackerel, and trout.

If you include meat in your endometriosis-relief program, I recommend using it in moderate amounts (6 ounces or less per day). Most Americans eat much more protein than is healthy. Excessive amounts of protein are difficult to digest and stress the kidneys. Except for fish, meat is also a main source of unhealthy saturated fats, which puts you at higher risk of heart disease and cancer.

Instead of using meat as your only source of protein, I recommend that you increase your intake of grains, beans, raw seeds, and nuts, which contain protein as well as many other important nutrients. For many years I have recommended that my patients use meat in smaller serving sizes and an ingredient for casseroles, stir-fries, and soups.

I also recommend buying the meat of organic, range-fed animals; this reduces the exposure to pesticides, antibiotics, and hormones. If you find meat difficult to digest, you may be deficient in hydrochloric acid. Try taking a small amount of hydrochloric acid with every meat-containing meal to see if your digestion improves.

Oils. You can use vegetable oils in small amounts for cooking, stir-frying, and sautéing. When you do, select an oil like olive oil or macadamia nut oil that contains healthy monounsaturated fat. These oils are also heart healthy, which is a great additional benefit and promote beautiful, shiny skin and hair.

Flaxseed oil, which is notable for its beautiful golden color and delicious nutty flavor, can be used to enhance the flavor of rice, steamed vegetables, toast, popcorn, and many other foods. Many of my patients use it as a butter substitute. However, you cannot cook with flax oil because it is very perishable, sensitive to heat, light, and oxygen. Instead, you must first cook the food, then add the flax oil just before serving. Keep flax oil tightly capped and refrigerated. All oils should be cold-pressed to help ensure freshness and purity. Keep your oils refrigerated to avoid rancidity.

Foods to Avoid with Endometriosis

If you have endometriosis, you should avoid or use only limited amounts of the foods described in this section. You will also notice that some of these foods are recognized as being high-stress or unhealthy foods for the body in general.

Dairy Products. Dairy products such as cheese, yogurt, milk, and cottage cheese should be avoided by women with endometriosis. Because dairy products have traditionally been touted as one of the four basic food groups, this information may be a surprise. Dairy products are the main dietary source of arachidonic acid, the fat used by your body to produce muscle-contracting F2 Alpha prostaglandins. These prostaglandins can increase pelvic pain, cramps, and inflammation characteristic of endometriosis. By deleting all dairy products from the diet, the severity of menstrual pain and cramps can be decreased by as much as one-third to one-half within one to two menstrual cycles.

The high saturated fat content of many dairy products is a risk factor for excess estrogen levels in the body. Research studies have shown that vegetarian women eating a low fat, high fiber diet excrete two to three times more estrogen in their bowel movements and have 50 percent lower blood levels of estrogen than women eating a diet high in dairy and animal fats. Bacteria in the colon actually convert metabolites of cholesterol to forms of estrogen that can be reabsorbed from the digestive tract back into the body. This elevates the body's estrogen levels which is a trigger for endometriosis and accelerates the spread of the disease. High estrogen levels have also been linked to heavy menstrual bleeding, another common complaint of women with these problems.

Dairy products have many other unhealthy effects on a woman's body. Many people are allergic to dairy products or lack the enzymes to digest milk. The result can be digestive problems such as bloating, gas, and bowel changes, which intensify with menstruation. This intolerance to dairy products can hamper the absorption and assimilation of calcium.

Because dairy products are a risk factor for endometriosis, women who have depended on dairy products for their calcium intake naturally wonder about alternative sources. The many other good dietary sources of this essential nutrient include beans, peas, soybeans, sesame seeds, soup stock made from chicken or fish bones, and green leafy vegetables. For food preparation, rice, almond, coconut, soy, flaxseed, hemp and sunflower seed milk are excellent substitutes. You can also use a supplement containing calcium, magnesium, and vitamin D to make sure your intake is sufficient. Nondairy milks are available at health food stores and some supermarkets.

Wheat and Gluten-Containing Grains. While consuming whole grains has many health benefits, some women with endometriosis and other conditions like PMS may find that they are allergic to or intolerant of wheat. Most women are surprised by this discovery, since wheat is one of the staples of our culture and is eaten by most people at almost every meal. However, wheat contains a protein called gluten, which is highly allergenic and difficult for the body to break down, absorb, and assimilate. Women with wheat intolerance are prone to fatigue, depression, sinusitis, allergies, bloating, intestinal gas, and bowel changes.

It can also affect hormonal health and worsen estrogen dominance, aggravating the symptoms of endometriosis. In my clinical practice, I have observed how wheat (along with other foods) can trigger emotional symptoms and fatigue in PMS patients, especially during the week or two before the onset of menses.

If you suffer from any of these conditions, you should probably eliminate wheat from your diet and use the many gluten-free breads, breakfast cereals, bagels, English muffins, cookies and other flour based foods that are readily available in health food stores and many supermarkets. Oats and rye, which also contain gluten, should be eliminated along with wheat if your symptoms are moderate to severe.

I have found over the years that the least stressful grain for women with estrogen dominant related conditions like endometriosis are grains like brown rice, millet, quinoa, wild rice, amaranth and buckwheat. Gluten-free oats are available in health food stores and some supermarkets.

Buckwheat is not commonly eaten in our culture, so most women never develop an intolerance to it. Also, it is not in the same plant family as wheat and other grains. Other infrequently used grains such as wild rice, quinoa, and amaranth should be tried as well. These are available in health food stores in breads, crackers, pastas and cereals.

Whole grass and whole grain flours can be prepared in a variety of ways, including whole grain cereals, breads, crackers, pancakes, waffles, and pastas. They can also be sprouted and eaten raw. A wide variety of these grains and products are available both in supermarkets and natural food stores.

Fats. Saturated fats in general come from animal sources, and from a few vegetable sources such as palm oil. Like dairy products, they contain arachidonic acid, and therefore can intensify menstrual cramps by stimulating production of the muscle-contracting prostaglandins. Unfortunately, in the typical American diet, a large part of the calories come from fat. Most of this fat comes from unhealthy saturated sources such as dairy products and red meat. This diet promotes heavy menstrual bleeding in susceptible women. Excessive saturated fat intake is stressful to the liver, so the liver is less able to break down estrogen efficiently, leading to excess estrogen levels.

Saturated fat, primarily from animal sources, also puts women at high risk of heart disease and cancers of the breast, uterus and ovaries. Women on a high-fat diet also tend to accumulate excess weight more easily. Instead of foods high in saturated fats, eat more fruits, vegetables, grains, fish and poultry. As often as possible, eat fresh and homemade foods prepared with a minimum of fats and oils.

If you must eat packaged and processed foods, read the labels. Avoid those with a high fat content. Red meat should be used only in small amounts. Avoid or adapt recipes that call for large amounts of butter, cream, cheese, or other high-fat ingredients. Instead, flavor foods with garlic, onions, herbs, lemon juice, or olive oil (a monosaturated fat that doesn't increase your cholesterol level). Eat raw seeds and nuts rather than cooked ones (cooking alters the nature of the oils), and use them sparingly because of their high fat content.

Salt. Excessive salt intake can worsen the menstrual symptoms that frequently occur in women with endometriosis. Too much dietary salt can increase bloating and fluid retention, particularly in women who have coexisting PMS. Too much salt intake can also increase high blood pressure and is a risk factor in the development of osteoporosis in menopausal women.

Unfortunately, most processed food contains large amounts of salt. Frozen and canned foods are often loaded with salt. In fact, one frozen-food entree can contribute as much as one-half teaspoon of salt to your daily intake. Large amounts of salt are also commonly found in the American diet as table salt (sodium chloride), MSG (monosodium glutamate), and a variety of food additives. Fast foods such as hamburgers, hot dogs, french fries, pizza and tacos are loaded with salt and saturated fats.

Common foods such as canned soups, potato chips, cheese, olives, salad dressings, and ketchup (to name only a few) are also very high in salt. To make matters worse, many people add too much salt while cooking and seasoning their meals.

Women with endometriosis should avoid adding salt to their meals. For flavor, use seasonings like garlic, herbs, spices, and lemon juice. Avoid processed foods that are high in salt. Learn to read labels and look for the word sodium (salt). If it appears high on the list of ingredients, don't buy the product. Many items in health food stores are labeled "no salt added." Some supermarkets also offer "no added salt" foods in their diet or health food sections.

Alcohol. Women with endometriosis should avoid alcohol entirely or consume it only in small amounts. Like dairy products and saturated fats, alcohol is stressful to the liver and can affect the liver's ability to metabolize hormones, including estrogen, efficiently.

Excessive alcohol intake has been associated with both lack of ovulation and elevated estrogen levels, which can trigger the growth and spread of endometrial implants in susceptible women, worsening menstrual cramps and pain. It can also trigger heavy bleeding in estrogen-sensitive women with endometriosis.

Excessive estrogen can worsen the congestive symptoms of menstrual pain and cramps. Estrogen causes fluid and salt retention in the body. When levels are too high, the body can retain excessive amounts of fluid during the premenstrual and menstrual phases of the month.

Alcohol also depletes the body's B-complex vitamins and minerals such as magnesium by disrupting carbohydrate metabolism. Because minerals are important in regulating muscle tension, an alcohol-based nutritional deficiency can worsen muscle spasms at the time of menstruation. Depletion of magnesium and vitamin B-complex can also intensify menstrual fatigue and mood swings.

Though alcohol has a relaxing effect and can enhance the taste of food, I recommend that women with endometriosis avoid or limit its use, particularly in the early stages of treatment. This is even more important for women who have coexisting PMS. For these women, the use of alcohol can aggravate the PMS-related mood swings, irritability, and other symptoms.

If you entertain a great deal and enjoy social drinking, try using non-alcoholic beverages. A nonalcoholic cocktail such as mineral water with a twist of lime or lemon or a dash of bitters is a good substitute. Light wine and beer—in small amounts—have a lower alcohol content than hard liquor, liqueurs, and regular wine.

Sugar. Like alcohol, sugar depletes the body's B-complex vitamins and minerals, which can worsen muscle tension and irritability as well as nervous tension and anxiety. Lack of certain B vitamins also hampers the liver's ability to handle fats, including the fat-based hormone estrogen. One particular B vitamin, B6, is needed for the production of beneficial types of prostaglandins that have relaxant and anti-inflammatory effects, both important for the treatment of endometriosis.

Unfortunately, sugar addiction is very common in our society in people of all ages. Many people use sweet foods to deal with their frustrations and other upsets. As a result, most Americans eat too much sugar—the average American eats 120 pounds each year.

Many convenience foods, such as salad dressing, ketchup and relish, contain high levels of both sugar and salt. Sugar is the main ingredient in soft drinks and in desserts such as candies, cookies, cakes and ice cream. Highly sugared foods also lead to tooth loss through tooth decay and gum disease. Of even greater significance is the fact that excessive sugar intake can aggravate diabetes and blood sugar imbalances.

Try to satisfy your sweet tooth instead with healthier foods, such as fruit or grain-based desserts like oatmeal cookies made with fruit or honey. You will find that small amounts of these foods can satisfy your cravings. Instead of disrupting your mood and energy level, they actually have a healthful and balancing effect.

Caffeine. Coffee, black tea, soft drinks, and chocolate—all these foods contain caffeine, a stimulant that many women use to increase their energy level and alertness and decrease fatigue.

Caffeine is even used in many over-the-counter menstrual remedies that women with early-stage endometriosis often take for symptom relief. Unfortunately, caffeine has many negative effects on the body. For example, caffeine used in excess increases anxiety, irritability, and mood swings. This can be a real problem for women in whom PMS coexists with endometriosis.

Caffeine also depletes the body's stores of B-complex vitamins and essential minerals, so long-term use can increase endometriosis-related pain, cramps, and bleeding by disrupting both carbohydrate metabolism and healthy liver function. Many menopausal women also complain that caffeine increases the number of hot flashes. Coffee, black tea, chocolate, and caffeinated soft drinks all act to inhibit iron absorption, thus worsening anemia.

How to Substitute Healthy Ingredients in Recipes

Learning how to make substitutions for high-stress ingredients in recipes allows you to use your favorite recipes without compromising your health and well-being. Many recipes include ingredients that women with cramps need to avoid, like dairy products, salt, sugar, chocolate, and wheat. By eliminating the high-stress foods and replacing them with healthier ingredients, you can still make almost any recipe that you choose. I have recommended this technique for years to my patients, who have found with delight that they can still make their favorite dishes, but in much healthier versions.

Some women choose to totally eliminate the high-stress ingredients from a recipe. For example, you might make a pasta and tomato sauce, but eliminate the Parmesan cheese topping, or make a Greek salad without the feta cheese. Some of my patients even make pizza without cheese, layering tomato sauce and lots of vegetables on top of a pizza crust. In many cases, the high-stress ingredients are not necessary in order to make foods taste good. Always remember, they can worsen your symptoms.

If you want to retain a particular high-stress ingredient, you can substantially reduce the amount you use, while still retaining the flavor and taste. Most of us have palates jaded by too much salt, fat, sugar, and other flavorings. In many dishes, we taste only the additives and never really enjoy the delicious flavor of the foods themselves.

During the years that I have substituted low-stress ingredients in my cooking, I have come to enjoy the subtle taste of the dishes much more. Also, I find that my health and vitality continue to improve with the deletion of high-stress ingredients from my food. The following information tells how to substitute healthy ingredients in your own recipes. The substitutions are simple to make and should benefit your health greatly.

How to Substitute for Caffeinated Foods and Beverages

Drink substitutes for coffee and black tea. The best substitutes are the grain-based coffee beverages like Postum and Cafix. Some women find it difficult to discontinue coffee abruptly, because they suffer withdrawal symptoms such as headaches. If this is a concern for you, decrease your total coffee intake gradually to one-half to one cup per day. Use coffee substitutes for your other cups. This will help prevent withdrawal symptoms.

Use decaffeinated coffee or tea as a transition beverage. If you cannot give up coffee, you can start by substituting water-process decaffeinated coffee for the real thing. Then try to wean yourself from coffee altogether.

Use herbal teas for energy and vitality. Many women drink coffee for the pick-up they get from it. Those morning cups of coffee allow them to wake up and function through the day. Use green tea or ginger tea, instead. Green tea contains small amounts of caffeine that many women tolerate well unless they have a tendency towards anxiety and panic attacks. These teas are great herbal stimulant that will support your health. They are both available as tea bags. To make ginger tea, grate a few teaspoons of fresh ginger root into a pot of hot water. Boil and steep. Serve with honey.

Substitute carob for chocolate. Unsweetened carob tastes like chocolate but is far more nutritious. It is a member of the legume family and is high in calcium. You can purchase it in chunk form as a substitute for chocolate candy, or in a powder for baking or drinks. Be careful, however, not to overindulge; carob, like chocolate, is high in calories and fat. It should be considered a treat and a cooking aid to be used only in small amounts.

How to Substitute for Dairy Products

Decrease the amount of cheese you use in food preparation and cooking. If you must use cheese, decrease the amount by two-thirds or more so that it becomes a flavoring or garnish rather than a major source of fat and protein. You can often replace cheese in recipes with soft tofu. I have done this with lasagna, layering the lasagna noodles with tofu and tomato sauce and topping with melted soy, vegan or non-casein rice cheese for a delicious dish. The tofu, which is bland, takes on the taste of the tomato sauce. If you cannot give up milk products, try to use the lower-fat cheeses now available. Goat or sheep's milk cheese in small amounts can also replace cheese, because the fat they contain is more easily emulsified in the body.

Use soy, vegan or non casein rice cheese in food preparation and cooking. These are excellent substitutes for cow's milk cheese. They are lower in fat and salt, and the fat that it contains isn't saturated. Health food stores offer many brands in many different flavors, such as mozzarella, cheddar, American, and jack. You can use soy, vegan and non-casein rice cheese as cheese substitutes in sandwiches, salads, pizzas, lasagnas and casseroles. Vegan and rice cheese can be used if you are soy intolerant.

Replace milk in recipes. For cow's milk, substitute nondairy milks like rice, almond, coconut, hemp, flaxseed, sunflower or soy milk. These milk substitutes are widely available at natural food stores and in most supermarkets. Rice and almond milk are particularly good tasting and an extra benefit is that nondairy milks are good sources of calcium. I have had very good feedback over the years from my patients who use these milk substitutes for drinking, mixing with hot or cold cereals, cooking, and baking. In addition to milk, there are now nondairy, vegetarian-based butter substitutes, sour cream, cream cheese, and frozen desserts, all of which taste quite delicious.

Substitute flax oil for butter. Flax oil is the best substitute for butter that I have found. It is a golden, rich oil that looks and tastes quite a bit like butter. It is delicious on anything you'd normally top with butter—toast, rice, popcorn, steamed vegetables and potatoes. Flax oil is extremely high in essential fatty acids—the type of fat that is very healthy for a woman's body. Essential fatty acids help promote normal hormonal function. Flax oil is quite perishable because it is sensitive to heat and light, so keep it refrigerated. You can't cook with it—always cook the food first and then add the flax oil before serving. Use it on toast, popcorn, steamed vegetables, rice, pasta, and mashed potatoes. There are so many health benefits to flax oil that I recommend it highly. You can find it in health food stores.

How to Substitute for Salt

Substitute potassium-based products for table salt (sodium chloride). Potassium-based products, such as Morton's Salt Substitute, are much healthier and will not aggravate heart disease or hypertension.

Substitute powdered seaweeds like kelp or nori to season vegetables, grains, and salads. They are high in essential iodine and trace elements.

Use herbs instead of salt for flavoring. Their flavors are much more subtle and will help even the most jaded palates appreciate the taste of vegetables and meats.

Use low-sodium content liquid flavoring agents. Low-salt soy sauce and Bragg's Amino Acids, a liquid soybean-based flavoring agent, are delicious when used as salt substitutes in cooking. When added to soups, casseroles, stir-fries, a small amount provides intense flavoring.

How to Substitute for Wheat Flour

While consuming whole grains has many health benefits, some women with endometriosis and other women's health issues like fibroid tumors may find that they are allergic to or intolerant of wheat. Most women are surprised by this discovery, since wheat is one of the staples of our culture and is eaten by most people at almost every meal. However, wheat contains a protein called gluten, which is highly allergenic and difficult for the body to break down, absorb, and assimilate. Women with wheat intolerance are prone to fatigue, depression, sinusitis, allergies, bloating, intestinal gas, and bowel changes.

In my clinical experience, when women are nutritionally sensitive, wheat consumption can often worsen emotional symptoms and lower energy levels. I have observed how wheat (along with other foods) can trigger emotional symptoms, bloating and fatigue in PMS patients, especially during the week or two before the onset of menses. Many menopausal women tolerate wheat poorly because their digestive tracts are beginning to show the wear and tear of aging and don't produce enough enzymes to break down wheat easily.

Women with allergies often find that wheat intensifies nasal and sinus congestion, as well as fatigue. I also find that women with poor resistance and a tendency toward infections may need to eliminate wheat from their diets to boost their immune systems. Since wheat is leavened with yeast, it should also be avoided by women with candida.

Use gluten-free grains. If you suffer from any of these conditions, as well as dull aching, cramping and bloating with PMS, you should probably eliminate wheat from your diet. I have found over the years that the least stressful grain for women with endometriosis are grains like brown rice, millet, quinoa, wild rice, amaranth and buckwheat. For example, buckwheat is not commonly eaten in our culture, so most women never develop an intolerance to it. Also, it is not in the same plant family as wheat and other grains. Buckwheat is actually the fruit-like structure of the plant rather than a grass. Other grains such as wild rice, quinoa, and amaranth should be tried as well. These are available in health food stores in pastas and cereals.

I recommend that you and use the many gluten-free breads, breakfast cereals, bagels, English muffins, cookies, pasta and other flour based foods that are readily available in health food stores and many supermarkets. Oats and rye, which contain gluten, should be eliminated along with wheat if your symptoms are moderate to severe. Gluten-free oats are available in health food stores and some supermarkets.

How to Substitute for Sugar

Cut the amount of sweetener in your recipes by one-third to one-half. This can be done easily without changing the taste of most dishes. Americans tend to be addicted to sugar. Most of us grew up on highly sugared soft drinks, candy, and rich pastries—no wonder the incidence of diabetes is soaring among our population. I have found that as women decrease their sugar intake, most begin to really enjoy the subtle flavors of the foods they eat.

Substitute healthy sweetening agents. Xylitol and stevia are two of my favorites. Stevia is an herbal sweetener that is calorie free. Thus, it is helpful if you are on a weight loss program or don't want the extra calories found in other sweeteners such as sugar or honey. Because stevia contains no calories from sugar, it does not create imbalances in the blood sugar level. This is very beneficial if you suffer from hypoglycemia or diabetes.

Xylitol is a wonderful sweetener that gives a delicious flavor to baked goods, desserts and beverages without the health problems related to table sugar like diabetes, candida infections, overweight and tooth decay. Even better, xylitol is as sweet as sugar but has only two thirds the calories.

Xylitol is absorbed more slowly than sugar so is helpful for diabetes, has antibacterial and antifungal properties and helps promote healthy teeth and gums. It is also found naturally in guavas, pears, blackberries, raspberries, aloe vera, eggplant, peas, green beans and corn.

Substitute concentrated sweeteners. Concentrated sweeteners such as honey and maple syrup have a sweeter taste per quantity used than table sugar. Using these substitutes will enable you to cut down on the amount of sugar used. If you use a concentrated sweetener in place of sugar in an ordinary recipe, reduce the liquid content in the recipe by one-fourth cup. If no liquid is used in the recipe, add 3 to 5 tablespoons of flour for each three-fourths cup of concentrated sweetener.

Substitute fruit for sugar in pastries. In making muffins and cookies, you may want to try deleting sugar altogether and adding extra fruits and nuts. Many of my patients like to use apple sauce and bananas as sweeteners in baked goods to cut down the need for sugar.

How to Substitute for Alcohol

Use low-alcohol or nonalcoholic products for cooking. Substitute low-alcohol or nonalcoholic wine or beer when cooking or preparing sauces and marinades. You will retain much of the flavor that alcohol imparts and you'll decrease the stress factor substantially.

Use sparkling water for parties and social events. Many of us enjoy holding a beverage while socializing. Instead of alcoholic beverages like wine, hard liquor or mixed drink, consider sparkling water with a twist of lemon or lime. A splash of bitter is also excellent. Or, combine sparkling water with a little fruit juice for a festive drink.

Substitutes for Common High-Stress Ingredients

¾ cup sugar	¾ cup xylitol
	½ cup honey
	¼ cup molasses
	½ cup maple syrup
	½ ounce barley malt
	1 cup apple butter
	2 cups apple juice
1 cup milk	1 cup soy, rice, flaxseed, hemp, coconut or almond milk
1 tablespoon butter	1 tablespoon flax oil (must be used raw and unheated)
½ teaspoon salt	1 tablespoon miso
	½ teaspoon potassium chloride salt substitute
	½ teaspoon Mrs. Dash, Spike
	½ teaspoon herbs (basil, tarragon, oregano, etc.)
1 ½ cups cocoa	1 cup powdered carob
1 square chocolate	¾ tablespoon powdered carob
1 tablespoon coffee	1 tablespoon decaffeinated coffee
	1 tablespoon Postum, Cafix, or other grain-based coffee substitute; green tea or ginger tea
4 ounces wine	4 ounces light wine
8 ounces beer	8 ounces near beer
1 cup white flour	1 cup barley flour (pie crust)
	1 cup rice flour (cookies, cakes, breads)

Healthy Food Shopping List

Vegetables

Beets	Eggplant	Radicchio
Bok choy	Garlic	Radishes
Broccoli	Green beans	Rutabagas
Brussels sprouts	Horseradish	Sauerkraut
Cabbage	Kale	Spinach
Carrots	Lettuce	Squash
Cauliflower	Mustard greens	Sweet potatoes
Celery	Okra	Tomatoes
Chard	Onions	Turnips
Cilantro	Parsley	Turnip greens
Collard	Parsnips	Watercress
Cucumbers	Peas (all varieties)	Yams
Dandelion greens	Potatoes	

Legumes	**Whole Grains**	**Seeds and Nuts**
Adzuki	Amaranth	Almonds
Black	Barley	Cashews
Black-eyed peas	Brown rice	Filberts
Cannellini	Buckwheat	Flaxseeds
Fava	Corn	Macadamia
Garbanzo	Millet	Pecan
Kidney	Oatmeal	Pumpkin seeds
Lentils	Quinoa	Sesame seeds
Navy	Rye	Sunflower seeds
Red		Walnuts
Soy: tofu, tempi		
Turtle beans		

Healthy Food Shopping List (continued)

Fruits
Acai berries
Apples
Avocado
Bananas
Berries
Blueberries
Raspberries
Strawberries
Coconuts
Goji berries
Kiwi
Noni
Olives
Pomegranates
Pears
Seasonal

Sweeteners
Brown rice syrup
Honey
Maple syrup
Molasses
Stevia
Xylitol

Beverages
Coconut water
Grain based coffee
substitute
Herbal tea
Green tea
Water

Meats
Fish
Free-range poultry
Game meat
Organic lean red meat
Seafood (in
moderation)

Oils
Flax
Macadamia
Olive
Safflower
Sesame
Walnut

Foods from Other Cultures
Gomasio
Jicama
Miso
Seaweed (like kelp,
dulse, nori, wakane)
Tamari soy sauce
Umeboshi plums

Dairy Substitutes
Hemp milk
Nut milk
Rice milk
Soy milk
Soy, coconut, almond,
rice or hemp cheeses,
cream cheese, yogurt,
and frozen desserts
*Avoid all soy products
containing
hydrogenated oil.

Herbs & Spices
Basil
Black pepper
Cayenne pepper
Chamomile
Chili pepper, dried
Cilantro
Cinnamon, ground
Cloves
Coriander
Cumin
Dill
Ginger
Licorice
Mustard seeds
Oregano
Peppermint
Poppy
Rosemary
Sage
Tarragon
Thyme
Turmeric

5

Menus, Meal Plans and Recipes

This chapter addresses the enjoyable subject of meal planning and dining. As I discussed in chapter 4, you can benefit greatly from eliminating certain high-stress foods that promote estrogen levels that are too high or trigger inflammation in order to gain symptom relief. Happily, a therapeutic diet can be just as delicious and pleasurable to the senses. With my endometriosis relief diet, not only are the foods delicious and enjoyable to eat, but you will gain the tremendous benefit of reduction of your endometriosis symptoms as well as improved health and well-being.

Upon learning the importance of diet and nutrition, most of my patients have asked me for specific menus, meal plans, and recipes to help them implement their own self-care programs. Unfortunately, very few specific resources are available. Most cookbooks do not adequately address a woman's needs for specific nutrients when they are suffering from endometriosis. Many contain recipes that are too high in the nutrients that can worsen cramps and inflammation such as animal fats, dairy products, chocolate, sugar, alcohol and salt.

Some nutrition-conscious cookbooks do -present low-calorie "light dishes" that eliminate the high-stress ingredients, but still don't give women with endometriosis the therapeutic levels of specific nutrients they need. As a result, I've developed these resources to best help you gain relief from this condition.

This chapter contains menus and recipes that I have created for my patients with very beneficial therapeutic results. No one diet fits the needs of all different body types. Because of this I have included menus and delicious recipes for women who prefer a vegetarian emphasis, high carbohydrate diet as well as dishes and entrees for women who feel their best on a high protein, meat based diet. All of these meal plans and recipes contain ingredients most suitable for women with endometriosis. In addition, the high stress ingredients that can worsen your symptoms have been eliminated.

Because many women lead busy lives and have many demands on their time, I've devised recipes that are quick and easy to prepare. I have found that anything too complicated doesn't work for either many of my patients. Best of all, these recipes are delicious as well as healthful. I hope that you find trying these new dishes to be a delightful adventure as well.

Breakfast Menus

These breakfast menus have been developed to help reduce and prevent symptoms of endometriosis. All the dishes contain high levels of the essential nutrients that women with these problems need; the recipes call for no high-stress ingredients. You can use these as idea generators for your own meal planning.

Breakfast has been one of the easiest meals for my patients to restructure along healthier lines. It tends to be a smaller and simpler meal. You may want to make healthful dietary changes in your breakfast first and then move on to lunch and dinner.

Flax shake with protein powder
and fresh fruit
~~~~~~~~~~~~~

Rice and flaxseed pancakes
Banana
Vanilla nondairy milk
~~~~~~~~~~~~~

Millet cereal with raisins and
cinnamon
Nondairy yogurt
Chamomile tea
~~~~~~~~~~~~~

Blueberry and spirulina smoothie
~~~~~~~~~~~~~

Oatmeal with raspberries
Chamomile tea
~~~~~~~~~~~~~

Nondairy yogurt with granola
and ground flaxseed
Peppermint tea
~~~~~~~~~~~~~

Scrambled eggs and turkey
bacon
Ginger tea
~~~~~~~~~~~~~

Omelette with chicken sausage
Roasted grain beverage (coffee
substitute)
~~~~~~~~~~~~~

Lunch and Dinner Menus

Here is a variety of menus you can choose from when planning your meals. You can use these menu plans or as idea generators to fit your own taste and needs. These dishes contain many nutritious and healthful ingredients for endometriosis relief. Use these menus as helpful guidelines throughout the entire month. Your nutritional status on a day-by-day basis determines in part how likely you are to have endometriosis symptoms. These dishes should help to diminish the severity of your symptoms because they eliminate high-stress foods.

Soup Meals
Split pea soup
Corn muffins
Fresh applesauce
~~~~~~~~~~~~~~~

Chicken and wild rice soup
Cole slaw
Millet bread with flax oil
~~~~~~~~~~~~~~~

Vegetable soup with brown rice
Steamed kale
Baked potato with flax oil
Apple slices
~~~~~~~~~~~~~~~

Lentil soup
Herbed brown rice
Broccoli with lemon
~~~~~~~~~~~~~~~

Tomato soup
Potato salad with low-fat mayonnaise
Celery and carrot sticks
~~~~~~~~~~~~~~~

Salad Meals
Spinach salad with turkey bacon or tofu
Corn muffins with flax oil
Orange slices
~~~~~~~~~~~~~~~

Beet salad with goat cheese
Rice crackers with fresh fruit preserves
~~~~~~~~~~~~~~~

Romaine salad with grilled salmon
Gluten-free bread and olive oil dip
~~~~~~~~~~~~~~~

Low-fat potato salad
Cole slaw
Hard boiled eggs
Melon slices
~~~~~~~~~~~~~~~

Mixed Vegetable Salad with Kidney Beans
Baked yam

Meat Meals

Poached salmon with lemon
Herbed brown rice
Steamed carrots with honey
~~~~~~~~~~~~~~~

Roasted chicken with herbs
Baked potato with flax oil
Broccoli with lemon
~~~~~~~~~~~~~~~

Broiled trout with dill
Mixed green salad with vinaigrette
Green peas and onions
Apple slices
~~~~~~~~~~~~~~~

Grilled shrimp with olive oil and
lemon
Wild rice
Steamed kale
~~~~~~~~~~~~~~~

One-Dish Vegetable Meals

Vegetarian tacos with black beans,
brown rice, avocados, tomatoes,
lettuce and low-salt salsa
~~~~~~~~~~~~~~~

Stir-fry with mixed vegetables,
brown rice and tofu
Orange slices
~~~~~~~~~~~~~~~

Pasta with tomato sauce, broccoli,
carrots, olive oil and garlic
Green salad with vinaigrette
~~~~~~~~~~~~~~~

Hummus dip
Eggplant dip (babaganoush)
Mixed raw vegetable slices
including carrots, red bell peppers,
and radishes
~~~~~~~~~~~~~~~

Brown rice and almond tabouli
Mixed olives
Melon slices
~~~~~~~~~~~~~~~

Breakfast Recipes

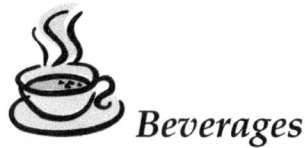 *Beverages*

These drinks are made with therapeutic herbal teas, power smoothies that are rich in fruits, raw seeds, nuts, protein powder, green foods and nondairy milk that are recommended for preventing and treating your symptoms. The ingredients contain high levels of essential nutrients that help regulate your hormonal balance and relax tension in the muscles of the pelvis and lower extremities. You can enjoy these beverages throughout the month, and not just during your symptom time, as their high mineral and other nutrient content is beneficial for the entire body.

Relaxant Herb Tea   **Serves 2**

2 cups water
1 teaspoon chamomile leaves
1 teaspoon peppermint leaves
1 teaspoon honey (if desired)

Bring the water to a boil. Place herbs in water and stir. Turn heat to low and simmer for 15 minutes.

Peppermint and chamomile are both muscle relaxants and antispasmodic herbs, so they can provide relief of pain and cramping caused by endometriosis. They also help calm the mood.

Ginger Tea   **Serves 4**

Ginger makes a warming, delicious tea and is beneficial to your circulation. It is also a powerful anti-inflammatory herb. If the tea is too strong add more water.

5 cups water
3 tablespoons ginger coarsely chopped
½ lemon (optional)
Honey (or other sweetener, to taste)

Add ginger to the water in a cooking pot. Bring to a boil and then turn heat to low. Steep for 15 or 20 minutes. Squeeze lemon into tea and serve with honey or your favorite sweetener.

Blueberry Coconut Smoothie   **Serves 2**

1 cup coconut water
⅔ cup blueberries – fresh or frozen
1 heaping tablespoon raw coconut flour
1 heaping tablespoon raw almonds (10-15)
1 banana, sliced

Combine all ingredients in a blender. Puree until smooth and serve.

Raspberry Flax Smoothie   **Serves 2**

This creamy smoothie makes a great breakfast. Flaxseed oil one is my favorite foods. It is both delicious and rich in healthy omega-3 fatty acids. It also adds extra creaminess to the smoothie.

1 cup rice milk
⅔ cup raspberries – fresh or frozen
1 heaping tablespoon rice protein powder
1 tablespoon flaxseed oil
2 bananas, sliced

Combine all ingredients in a blender. Puree until smooth and serve.

Delicious Green Drink   Serves 1

½ cup Concord grape juice
¼ cup water
1 tablespoon ground flaxseed
½ teaspoon chlorella powder
½ teaspoon spirulina powder

Mix all ingredients together in a glass or puree in a blender.

Blueberry and Greens Shake   Serves 2

This drink is a powerhouse of nutrients! The chlorella and spirulina are highly beneficial green foods. They are rich in nutrients like beta-carotene and help to detoxify the liver. They are readily available at health food stores.

1 cup nondairy milk
⅔ cup blueberries – fresh or frozen
2 tablespoons protein powder
½ teaspoon chlorella
½ teaspoon spirulina
Sprinkle of Truvia (optional)

In a blender puree the nondairy milk and blueberries. Add the rest of the ingredients and blend well.

Simple Flax Smoothie   Serves 2

Flaxseed is not only a tasty addition to smoothies but it is also very nutritious. Flaxseed is high in essential fatty acids, calcium, magnesium, and potassium.

1 cup vanilla nondairy milk
2 tablespoons ground flaxseed
1 banana

Combine all ingredients in a blender. Blend until smooth and serve.

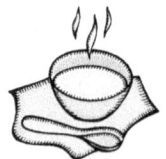 *Healthy, Quick Breakfasts*

Most American breakfasts include wheat and dairy products, such as yogurt, wheat toast, wheat cereal with milk, sweet rolls, and other wheat-based pastries. As I explained in Chapter 4, dairy products and wheat can worsen the symptoms of endometriosis and PMS (which often occurs concurrently).

I have included in this section both whole grain, carbohydrate based entrees as well as protein-rich dishes, depending on the type of diet that makes you feel your best. Both types of entrees, however, will benefit endometriosis symptoms by eliminating wheat and dairy products at breakfast.

The whole grain dishes are based on ground flaxseed, soy, and gluten-free grains, all of which can be useful in reducing your symptoms. Gluten is the protein found in wheat that can trigger symptoms of bloating, digestive disturbances, and fatigue. The protein-rich entrees have been created using eggs and healthy breakfast meats,

Quinoa Cereal with Raspberries   **Serves 2**

1 ½ cups cooked quinoa
1 cup nondairy milk
½ cup raspberries
2 teaspoons honey or other sweetener

Combine quinoa and nondairy milk in a saucepan. Simmer for 5 minutes. Stir in honey and garnish with raspberries.

Quinoa with Prunes   **Serves 2**

This is one of my all-time favorite hot cereals. The plums are delicious and add a nice texture. Quinoa is a small, protein rich grain. When cooked the grains are small and fluffy. I recommend making a pot of quinoa the night before.

1 ½ cups cooked quinoa
1 cup nondairy milk
4-6 dried prunes, chopped
2 tablespoons flaxseed oil
2 teaspoons xylitol, honey, or maple syrup (if using unsweetened milk)
Pinch of salt (optional)

In a saucepan combine quinoa, nondairy milk, salt, and dried plums. Heat thoroughly and simmer on low heat for 5-10 minutes until plums have softened. Serve with flaxseed oil and sweetener.

Maple Cinnamon Oatmeal   **Serves 2**

1 cup gluten-free quick oats
1 ¾ cups water
1-2 tablespoons flaxseed oil
2 teaspoons maple syrup
Pinch of cinnamon (to taste)
Pinch of salt

Boil water in a saucepan. Add gluten-free oats and reduce to medium heat. Cook for one minute and stir. Cover, and remove oatmeal from heat. Serve in 2-3 minutes.

Stir in maple syrup, flaxseed oil, cinnamon and salt.

Strawberries and Cream Oatmeal   Serves 2

1 cup gluten-free quick oats
½ cup strawberries, chopped
½ nondairy milk
1 ¼ cups water
1-2 tablespoons flaxseed oil
2 teaspoons honey or stevia
Pinch of salt (optional)

Bring water and nondairy milk to a boil in a saucepan. Add gluten-free oats and reduce to medium heat. Cook for one minute and stir. Cover, and remove oatmeal from heat. Serve in 2-3 minutes. Stir in sweetener, flaxseed oil, salt and top with strawberries.

Banana Nut Muffins   Makes 14-18

These moist muffins are a twist on the classic recipe using cashews instead of walnuts. Very tasty!

1½ cups rice flour
1 teaspoon baking powder
½ teaspoon baking soda
3 ripe bananas, mashed
¼ teaspoon cinnamon
6 packets of Truvia (¼ cup)
¼ cup honey
¼ cup safflower oil
¼ cup cashews, chopped

Preheat oven to 350 degrees. Mix all dry ingredients and wet ingredients separately. Combine and mix well. Fill muffin cups ⅔ with the batter.

Pumpkin Muffins Makes 14-18 muffins

1½ cups rice flour
½ teaspoon baking powder
½ teaspoon baking soda
1 cup pumpkin
1 teaspoon cinnamon
¼ teaspoon nutmeg
¼ cup chopped almonds (optional)
3 tablespoons molasses
3 tablespoons safflower oil
½ cup raisins
2 eggs
½ cup nondairy milk
1 teaspoon vanilla extract
Pinch of salt

Preheat oven to 400 degrees. Line a muffin tin with paper muffin cups.

Combine all dry ingredients and mix thoroughly. In a separate bowl beat the two eggs and then combine the remainder of the wet ingredients. Add the wet ingredients to the dry and mix thoroughly.

Fill muffin cups ⅔ with the batter. Cook for 18-20 minutes or until thoroughly cooked.

Flaxseed Pancakes   **Makes 8 pancakes (serves 2-4)**

Xylitol is an excellent sugar substitute for cooking and baking that can be found at most health food stores. Xylitol is easy to use because it has a 1:1 ratio with sugar. Yet, this product has 40% fewer calories than sugar and is beneficial for your teeth and gums.

1 cup gluten-free flour
1 cup unsweetened rice milk
1 egg
2 tablespoons xylitol
1 tablespoon ground flaxseed
1 teaspoon baking powder
½ teaspoon baking soda
¼ teaspoon salt
3 tablespoons almond oil, keeping 1 tbsp. for cooking
Maple syrup (optional)
Fruit jam (optional)

Mix the dry and wet ingredients in separate bowls. Combine all the ingredients and mix thoroughly. Cook on medium heat and use a small amount of oil to grease the pan if needed. When pancakes bubble in the center flip and cook for 1-2 minutes until cooked thoroughly. Serve with maple syrup or all-fruit jam. Delicious!

Egg and Sausage Scramble   **Serves 2**

4 eggs
4 turkey breakfast sausages
2 slice of gluten-free toast
Salt and pepper (optional)
2 teaspoons olive oil
Serve with ½ cup applesauce

Warm a frying pan on medium heat and add olive oil. Beat egg gently in a small bowl and set aside. Chop the sausages into small pieces - this will help them to cook faster. Add sausages to the pan and cook for several minutes until sausages are brown. Turn heat to low and add eggs to the pan and scramble with the sausage. Add a pinch of salt and pepper. Serve with toast and applesauce.

Bake for 20-25 minutes until cooked through.

Mushroom Onion Scramble   **Serves 2**

The mushrooms and onion give this egg scramble a great texture. The water helps make the eggs fluffier.

4 eggs
1 tablespoon water
¼ onion
2-3 mushrooms
1 tablespoon olive oil
Salt and pepper (optional)

Dice the mushrooms and onion. Next, beat the 4 eggs together with 1 tablespoon water. Preheat the frying pan on medium heat and add 1 tablespoon olive oil. Add onion and mushroom and cook for about 3 minutes until onions are translucent and add eggs. Let sit for about 30 second and then start to scramble with your spatula. Add a pinch of salt and pepper and serve.

Spinach and Tomato Scramble   **Serves 2**

The Parmesan cheese adds a delightful saltiness and tang to this dish.

4 eggs, beaten
1 tablespoon water
2 tablespoons diced onion
¼ tomato, chopped
12 spinach leaves, chopped
1 tablespoon olive oil
Salt and pepper (optional)
Parmesan cheese - or soy Parmesan (optional)

Beat the 4 eggs together with 1 tablespoon water. Preheat the frying pan on medium heat and add 1 tablespoon olive oil. Add onion and cook for about 3 minutes until onions are translucent. Next add eggs, spinach and tomato. Let sit for about 15 seconds and then start to scramble with your spatula. Sprinkle on a small amount of Parmesan cheese, add a pinch of salt and pepper and serve.

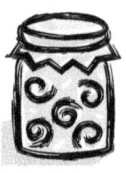 *Spreads and Sauces*

These spreads and sauces contain highly concentrated levels of ingredients that help to relax endometriosis-related pain and muscle tension and help to relieve congestion. Serve with rice cakes, crackers, corn bread, or even spread on a banana for a delicious treat.

Fresh Applesauce   **Serves 2**

2 ½ apples
½ cup fresh apple juice
½ teaspoon cinnamon
½ teaspoon ginger

Peel apples and cut into quarters; remove cores. Combine all ingredients in a food processor. Blend until smooth.

Sesame-Tofu Spread   **Serves 4**

¼ cup soft tofu
¼ cup raw sesame butter
¼ cup honey

Combine all ingredients in a blender. Serve with rice cakes or crackers.

Lunch and Dinner Recipes

These high-nutrient, healthful lunch and dinner dishes are designed to help prevent and relieve your symptoms. The ingredients do not include red meat, dairy products, or wheat, all of which can worsen your symptoms. Mix and match these dishes as you please. You might combine soups and salads or whole grains, legumes and vegetables for a complete vegetarian emphasis or meat-based meal, depending on your needs for carbohydrates and protein.

The main course dishes are all extremely healthful for women with endometriosis. You can enjoy these dishes particularly during the second half of your menstrual cycle when your symptoms are worse, but for optimal health and well-being, I recommend their use all month long.

 *Soups*

Split Pea Soup   **Serves 4**

¾ cup split peas
5 cups low-sodium chicken broth
¾ cup carrot, chopped
¾ cup onion, diced
Tamari soy sauce – to taste (optional)

Bring the water to a boil and add the split peas, onion, carrots, and chicken broth. Reduce heat to low and simmer for 50 minutes – 1 hour, stirring occasionally. If water begins to cook off add up to an extra cup of water. Add a dash of tamari soy sauce for a saltier flavor.

Black Bean Soup   Serves 4

This recipe is easy and makes a delicious, filling soup.

1 can black beans (14 ounce), rinsed
5 cups low-sodium vegetable broth
1 cup onion, diced
⅔ cup carrot, chopped
⅔ cup red pepper, chopped
¼ teaspoon cumin
Tamari soy sauce – to taste (optional)

Bring the water to a boil and add all ingredients. Reduce heat to low and simmer for 30 minutes, stirring occasionally. If water begins to cook off add up to an extra cup of water. Add a dash of tamari soy sauce for a saltier flavor.

Chicken Rice Soup   Serves 4-6

Few things make me feel better than a bowl of homemade chicken rice soup. I have an easy tip to add extra flavor to your soup: If you used the meat from a roasted, skin-on chicken you can add some of the skin to the soup while it is cooking. This will add depth and richness to your soup. Remove the skin when the soup has finished cooking.

6 cups low-sodium chicken broth
⅔ cup carrot
1 cup celery, diced
1 cup cooked chicken, diced
⅔ cup onion, diced
⅔ cup brown rice, cooked
Tamari soy sauce – to taste (optional)

Bring water to a boil and add all ingredients. Reduce heat to low and simmer for 30 minutes, stirring occasionally. If water begins to cook off add up to an extra cup of water. Add a dash of tamari soy sauce for a saltier flavor.

Butternut Squash Soup   **Serves 4**

This soup has been a long-time favorite of mine. I adore the light, creamy texture. Adding maple syrup enhances the natural sweetness of the squash.

½ onion, diced
1 cup low-sodium chicken broth
2 cups pureed butternut squash - fresh or frozen (fresh is preferred)
½ teaspoon cinnamon
1½ cups nondairy milk
2 teaspoons maple syrup
1 tablespoon safflower oil
½-¾ teaspoon salt

In a large saucepan heat the oil on medium heat. Add the onion and cook until translucent. Add the butternut squash, chicken broth, cinnamon and salt. Mix well and simmer for 5 minutes. Add nondairy milk and maple syrup. Simmer on low heat for ten minutes. Stir frequently while cooking the soup. *Optional*: To make extra creamy, blend the soup when it has finished cooking. Wait for the soup to cool before blending.

Salads

Classic Spinach Salad   Serves 4

My tip for cooking great turkey bacon is to cook it on medium-low heat. It takes a few extra minutes but is definitely worth it!

1 bunch of spinach, approximately 6 cups
4 slices of turkey bacon, cooked crisp and crumbled
2 eggs, sliced or chopped
½ cup red pepper, chopped
¼ red onion, sliced very thin
¾ cup mushrooms, sliced thin
Balsamic Vinaigrette Dressing

In a large bowl place the turkey bacon, egg, red pepper, onion, and mushrooms on top of the spinach. Before serving, add the dressing and toss the salad.

Zingy Watercress Salad   Serves 4

I enjoy the refreshing bitterness of watercress. This salad pairs well with green apple. Watercress has a strong flavor and a little goes a long way.

1 cup watercress, coarsely chopped
4 cups butter lettuce (or other soft lettuce), coarsely chopped
2 teaspoons scallions, finely chopped
½ green apple, chopped
1 ounce goat cheese, crumbled
Vinaigrette dressing

In a large bowl toss the watercress, butter lettuce, green onion, and apple together with the vinaigrette dressing (to taste). On top of the salad crumble the goat cheese.

Potato Salad with Vinaigrette Dressing   **Serves 4-6**

10-12 small red potatoes, cut into bite size pieces (about 2 cups)
2 tablespoons diced celery
2 tablespoons diced red onion
2 tablespoons diced red pepper
1 heaping tablespoon diced water chestnuts
1 hardboiled egg, yolk removed
Vinaigrette dressing (to taste)

Steam the potatoes for 15-20 minutes or until fork tender and let cool. Chop up all the vegetables into small pieces and set aside. Chop egg white and set aside. Toss with your favorite vinaigrette dressing.

Scrumptious Veggie Salad   **Serves 4-6**

This is one of my favorite salads! It pairs wonderfully with soups and sandwiches

1 head red lettuce, chopped into bite size pieces
1 large tomato, chopped
2 green onions, sliced
6 mushrooms, sliced
¾ cup kidney beans – canned works well
1 avocado, sliced
¼ cup sunflower seeds
Vinaigrette dressing (to taste)

Combine all ingredients except for avocado in a large salad bowl. Mix in Vinaigrette Dressing and top with avocado slices before serving.

Radicchio and Orange Salad **Serves 4-6**

This is a sophisticated and delicious salad. I love salads with "extras" such as fruit or a little bit of goat cheese.

6 cups salad greens
½ radicchio, sliced thin
¼ red onion, sliced very thin
3 ounces goat cheese
1 medium sized orange, peeled and cut into bite size segments
Orange vinaigrette

In a large bowl combine salad greens, radicchio, onion, and oranges. Pour vinaigrette, to taste, over salad and toss. Add goat cheese before serving.

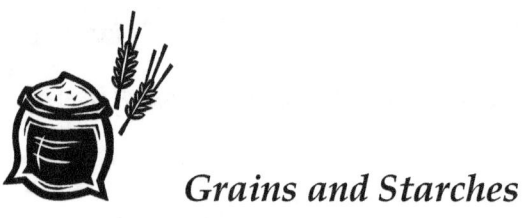 *Grains and Starches*

Wild Rice
Serves 2

⅔ cup wild rice
2 ½ cups water
½ teaspoon salt

Wash rice with cold water. Combine all ingredients in a cooking pot and bring to a rapid boil. Turn flame to low, cover, and cook without stirring (about 45 minutes) until rice is tender but not mushy. Uncover and fluff with a fork. Cook an additional 5 minutes, and then serve.

Kasha
Serves 4

1 cup kasha (buckwheat groats)
3 ¼ cups water
Pinch salt

Bring ingredients to a boil, lower heat, and simmer for 25 minutes or until soft. The grains should be fluffy, like rice.

For breakfast, blend in blender with water until creamy. Add almond milk, sesame milk, or sunflower milk, and cinnamon, apple butter, raisins, or berries.

Delicious Baked Sweet Potato
Serves 4

4 sweet potatoes
1 teaspoon olive oil
1 tablespoon flax oil for each potato

Preheat oven to 400° F. Wash the potatoes, then rub with olive oil. Bake for 45 to 60 minutes, or until soft when pierced with a fork. Garnish with flax oil. Honey, maple syrup, or chopped raw pecans may also be used.

Baked Potato   **Serves 4**

4 russet or Idaho potatoes
2 teaspoons olive oil
1 tablespoon flax oil for each potato

Preheat oven to 400° F. Wash the potatoes, rub them with olive oil, and bake for 45 to 60 minutes, or until soft when pierced with a fork. Garnish with flax oil. Other garnishes can include chopped green onions, soy cheese, and salsa.

 *Vegetables*

Kale with Lemon   Serves 4

Kale is one of my favorite vegetables and it also has terrific health benefits for women since it is a good source of calcium and other essential nutrients like lutein that supports the health of your eyes.

1 bunch of kale
1 lemon, cut into quarters
Soy sauce

Rinse kale well and remove stems. Steam for 5-6 minutes or until leaves wilt and are tender. Dress lightly with soy sauce and lemon juice.

Simple Steamed Cabbage   Serves 4

1 small head cabbage, quartered
1 teaspoon chopped parsley
1 teaspoon olive oil
Pinch of salt (optional)

Steam cabbage until tender. Sprinkle with olive oil and parsley.

Jessica's Favorite Broccoli   Serves 4

1 pound broccoli
1 tablespoons flax oil
Pinch of salt (optional)
Squeeze of lemon

Cut the broccoli into small florets; steam until tender. Squeeze lemon juice over broccoli and add the flax oil. Mix and serve.

Cauliflower with Flax Oil　　　　　　　　　　　　　　　　**Serves 4**

1 medium head cauliflower
2 tablespoons flax oil
Pinch of salt (optional)

Break the cauliflower into small florets. Steam until tender. Toss with flax oil and salt.

Roasted Rosemary Potatoes　　　　　　　　　　　　　　**Serves 4-6**

I love roasted potatoes! This is a wonderful potato recipe that I like to make when I serve roasted chicken.

4 cups red potatoes – about 4 or 5 large red potatoes
1 tablespoon dried rosemary, crushed
3 tablespoons of olive oil
2 garlic cloves, minced
¼ teaspoon black pepper (optional)
Pinch of salt

Preheat oven to 400 degrees. Cut potatoes into bite size pieces and put into plastic bag. Add olive oil, rosemary, garlic, and black pepper to bag. Close bag and shake to coat all of the potato pieces.

Line a baking tray with foil and put potatoes on to tray. Arrange evenly in one layer. Sprinkle salt onto potatoes and bake for 30-35 minutes until brown and cooked through. During cooking stir the potatoes once if desired.

Honey Carrots **Serves 4**

This is one of my favorite side dishes. The warm honey brings out the natural sweetness of the carrots.

3 cups carrots, sliced thin
1 teaspoon honey
1 teaspoon almond oil
Pinch of salt (optional)

Cut carrots into thin slices and steam for 6-8 minutes, or until tender. Using the same saucepan pour out the cooking water and on low heat add the honey and oil and mix well. Add carrots and mix all ingredients together. Add a pinch of salt before serving.

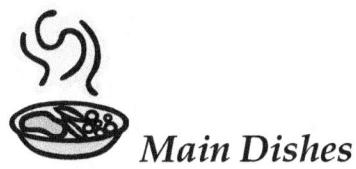 *Main Dishes*

Mega Greens Rice Bowl   **Serves 4**

This dish is a satisfying way to get a large serving of healthy greens. A delicious sauce is Organicville's Island Teriyaki (organicvillefoods.com). Their sauce is made with agave nectar instead of cane sugar.

4 cups kale, cut into bite size pieces (about ½ bunch)
3 cups baby bok choy, chopped
1 cup of white mushrooms, sliced
1 carrot, finely chopped
8 ounces of tofu, cubed
3 cups cooked brown rice - ¾ cup rice per person
Teriyaki sauce – soy sauce - gomasio

Steam the carrots for 4 minutes and then add the kale, bok choy, mushrooms, and tofu. Steam for 5 minutes. Serve in a deep bowl over rice with your choice of sauce.

Good sauces for this dish include teriyaki sauce and soy sauce. A little bit of lemon juice and gomasio also works well.

Baked Tofu Rice Bowl   Serves 4

Baked tofu has a rich, nutty flavor that I love. This recipe is fun but also very tasty and rich in healthy greens. I always make sure that the vegetables are cut into bite size pieces.

3 cups broccoli, chopped
3 cups baby bok choy, chopped
1 carrot, finely chopped
½ cup mushrooms, sliced
½ cup red pepper
Baked tofu
3 cups cooked brown rice - ¾ cup rice per person

Steam the carrots for 4 minutes and then add the broccoli, baby bok choy, mushrooms, and red pepper. Steam for 5 minutes. Serve in a deep bowl over rice with your choice of sauce. Layer a few pieces of baked tofu on top.

Summertime Veggie Pasta   Serves 4

This light pasta is one of my favorite dishes to eat during the summer. The pasta and sauce are light but filling. It's a dish that I love to share to share with friends.

1 box quinoa elbow pasta (8 ounce box)
½ onion, diced
2 cans Italian seasoned diced tomatoes
1 can garbanzo beans
1 carrot, shredded
1½ cups cooked Brussels sprouts or broccoli
½ teaspoon dried basil
2 teaspoons olive oil
⅛ teaspoon pepper
Pinch of salt (optional)

Cook pasta according to package directions. In a saucepan on medium heat add olive oil and onions. Sautee until onions are translucent. Add remainder of ingredients and bring to a simmer. Cook on low heat for 10 minutes. Combine the cooked noodles with the sauce.

Eggplant Parmesan   **Serves 4-6**

I love eggplant Parmesan. It is a rich and extremely delicious entree. This version, while wonderful, takes a little more time and has a few more steps than most of my entrees. Even though I use substitutions for the cheese, the dish is still very rich and I recommend saving it for a special occasion or party. You will wow your guests with how tasty it is! My favorite cheese alternative is by Follow Your Heart. Their products can be found in health food stores or at followyourheart.com

1 eggplant, cut into ⅓ - ½ inch slices (peeling is optional)
2 eggs, beaten
1 ¼ cups gluten-free bread crumbs
3 cups of pasta sauce, tomato and basil flavor
8 ounces of mozzarella cheese, shredded
¼ cup Parmesan or soy Parmesan cheese, grated
¼ cup olive oil - divided

Arrange the eggplant slices in a colander or on a rack placed over the sink. Sprinkle all of the slices generously with salt and let stand 30 minutes; the eggplant slices will release water. Rinse and pat dry. Next, dip each slice in the beaten egg and coat with breadcrumbs.

Heat a portion of the olive oil in a skillet over medium heat. Cook the eggplant until golden on each side, about 2-3 minutes. If necessary, reduce the heat to medium-low. Repeat until all of the eggplant is cooked.

Preheat the oven to 350°. Arrange half the eggplant slices on the bottom of a lightly oiled baking dish (a 9x9 or 9x12 pan works well). Spread half of the pasta sauce on top. Sprinkle with half of the mozzarella and half of the Parmesan cheese. Repeat with the next layer.

Bake 25-30 minutes or until mixture is bubbly.

Parmesan Chicken Pasta   **Serves 4**

This dish is a crowd pleaser that I often serve when I have friends over. The Parmesan cheese adds a delightful tanginess that rounds out the dish perfectly.

6 cups gluten-free pasta, cooked
1 ½ cups roasted chicken, cubed
¾ cup diced carrots
¾ cup diced red onion
½ onion, diced
1 small tomato, finely chopped
3 cups broccoli, chopped into bite size pieces
¾ cup chicken broth (recommended) or water
1 teaspoon dried basil
1 tablespoon olive oil
Soy Parmesan cheese or regular, grated
Generous pinch of pepper
Pinch of salt (optional)

In a frying pan on medium heat add the olive oil. Add the onion and sauté until onion begin to turn translucent. Add all vegetables except tomatoes and cook for 1-2 minutes. Add chicken broth, chicken, tomatoes, basil, and pepper. Turn heat to low, cover and simmer for 5-7 minutes or until broth has cooked down. Add more broth if needed.

Add the sauce to the pasta. Serve with soy Parmesan cheese.

Simple Broiled Tuna   **Serves 4**

4 fillets of tuna, 4 ounces each
2 teaspoons olive oil
Squeeze of lemon juice
Pinch of salt

Baste the tuna fillets with oil; then sprinkle with lemon juice. Place tuna in a broiler pan and broil until the level of doneness that you prefer (rare or well-done).

Simple Steamed Salmon   **Serves 4**

4 fillets of salmon, 4 ounces each
1 cup water
Squeeze of lemon

Combine water and lemon juice in a steamer. Place salmon fillets in streamer basket. Cook to the level of doneness that you prefer.

Turkey Bolognese   **Serves 2-4**

This dish cooks up quickly and is very satisfying. This is a versatile recipe. You can add all kinds of vegetables and it will taste great.

½ lb. ground turkey
2 cans of diced tomatoes
1 can tomato paste
½ onion, diced
1 carrot, diced
1 zucchini, diced
1 teaspoon basil
1 teaspoon oregano
1 tablespoon olive oil
¼ teaspoon salt (optional)
½ teaspoon black pepper (optional)
Water (optional)

Heat pan on medium and add olive oil. Add onion and sauté until translucent. Add turkey and all herbs and spices. Cook until turkey has browned and cooked thoroughly. Add tomatoes, tomato paste, carrots, and zucchini. Cook on low heat for 12-15 minutes. If sauce is too thick add a small amount of water until desired consistency is reached. Serve over brown rice spaghetti.

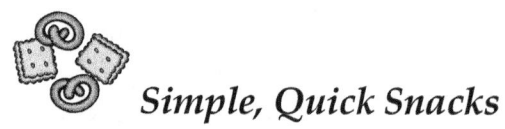 *Simple, Quick Snacks*

Trail Mix   **Makes ¾ cup**

¼ cup raw unsalted pumpkin seeds
¼ cup raw unsalted sunflower seeds
¼ cup raisins

Combine and store in a container in the refrigerator. This trail mix is very high in essential fatty acids, calcium, magnesium, and iron. I use it for a snack food to replace stressful and unhealthy sugar-based sweets and chocolate. It is a great mix to take on trips, and I eat it often for breakfast.

Rice Cakes with Nut Butter and Jam   **Serves 2**

4 unsalted rice cakes
2 tablespoons raw almond butter
2 tablespoons fruit preserves (no sugar added)

Spread rice cakes with almond butter and fruit preserves for a quick snack.

Herbal tea makes a good accompaniment.

Rice Cakes with Tuna Fish   **Serves 2**

4 unsalted rice cakes
4 ounces tuna fish
1 teaspoon low-calorie mayonnaise

Spread rice cakes with tuna fish and mayonnaise.

This is an excellent high-protein, high-carbohydrate snack.

Apple with Almond Butter   Serves 2

1 apple, sliced
1 tablespoon raw almond butter

Spread almond butter on thin apple slices.

Banana with Sesame Butter   Serves 2

1 banana, halved
1 tablespoon raw sesame butter

Spread sesame butter on each half of a ripe banana.

6

Vitamins, Minerals, Herbs and Essential Fatty Acids

Nutritional supplements can play an important role in the treatment and prevention of endometriosis. My program will help to dramatically reduce your symptoms of endometriosis through modifying two crucial hormonal and chemical pathways.

First, my program includes supplements that can help to balance your hormones and reduce estrogen levels by affecting estrogen production and metabolism at four crucial steps. These include reducing estrogen production by the ovaries and adrenal glands as well as interfering with estrogen's ability to bind to tissue receptors, especially to the pelvic organs like the ovaries and uterus. In addition, my supplement program also supports the breakdown and detoxification of estrogen by the liver and promotes its elimination from the body through the intestinal tract. The end result is less estrogen stimulating the growth of the endometriosis implants.

My nutritional supplement program will also help to increase your production of progesterone. This will help to counter the growth stimulating effects of estrogen on endometriosis implants.

Secondly, I discuss very effective supplements that will help to eliminate inflammation within your body. This is essential for the treatment of endometriosis since it is also a painful inflammatory condition. Nutritional supplements can greatly help to reduce the severity and spread of the inflammatory implants that are typical of this condition.

The end result of this combined approach can be a dramatic reduction in your symptoms of pain, cramping, irregular bleeding and can even assist in countering the infertility and difficulty conceiving that is often seen with endometriosis. My program has often saved my patients from needing to undergo a hysterectomy or the necessity to be on ovulation suppressing drugs. These medications have severe side-effects that cause a menopause like state of hormonal deficiency during the time of treatment with hot flashes and even bone loss.

I have been thrilled by the great benefits that I have seen with so many of my endometriosis patients who have followed my nutritional supplement program. The importance of nutrition in balancing estrogen levels, reducing inflammation, and relieving excessive menstrual bleeding, cramping and pain is also supported by medical research studies done at university centers and hospitals.

However, I do want to stress that the use of nutritional supplements must go hand in hand with a low-stress, healthful diet. It is not enough to take supplements and continue with poor dietary habits. It is important that you read and follow the dietary principals that I discuss in this book. Diet and the use of nutritional supplements need to go hand in hand for optimal healing. This is because diet alone can't provide the nutrient levels necessary for to control and heal endometriosis. The use of supplements can speed up and facilitate your return to vibrant health and well-being.

This chapter is divided into two sections. The first section discusses the role of vitamins, minerals and herbs for treating estrogen dominance and bringing estrogen and progesterone back into better balance. I also discuss nutritional supplements that are helpful for the relief of endometriosis related inflammation (**See the end of this chapter for a helpful summary chart).**

In the second section, I share with you a sample nutritional formula for endometriosis and give guidelines on how to use supplement products. There are also charts that list major food sources of each essential nutrient discussed.

As you read through this chapter, you will notice that in many sections, I have included several nutritional supplement options to help bring a crucial chemical step necessary for your hormonal health back into balance. I recommend that you read through the different options and choose those that most appeal to you. For example, in the first section, you may find that you are more drawn toward using soy foods and soy isoflavones for modulating estrogen production. However, if you don't tolerate or like soy, you may prefer to instead use flaxseed or citrus bioflavonoids to achieve the same positive result.

Decreasing Estrogen Dominance

Now, I want to summarize in more detail how to decrease estrogen dominance and increase progesterone production. Then we'll look more closely at each step in this process.

You can decrease estrogen production at both the adrenal level and the ovarian level by using weakly estrogenic herbs and nutrients to bind to key enzymes, thereby preventing the male hormones testosterone and androstenedione from being converted into estrogen. These enzymes are aromatase in the adrenals and estrogen synthetase in the ovaries. By blocking your body's own more potent estrogen from binding to the enzyme itself, you can hinder complete estrogen production from taking place. At the same time, you are providing the body with less potent, safer, and healthier estrogen-like chemicals from nutrients to support your body's needs during the transition into menopause.

At the same time, in order to effectively break down, metabolize, and eliminate estrogen from the body, you need to ensure that your liver, gallbladder, and intestinal tract are working properly and effectively. If these organs are not performing to optimum capacity, they cannot adequately metabolize and eliminate estrogen. Without proper deactivation of estrogen, there is more free-floating hormone circulating in your body.

This is how the whole system works: As estrogen goes through the detoxification process in your liver, it is inactivated by being bound to sulfuric and glucuronic acid and converted from the more potent form of estrogen—estradiol—to the less potent forms of estrone and estriol. This process of binding hormones with other chemicals makes them unable to attach to the specific hormone receptor sites within the cells. Once estrogen has been detoxified by the liver, it is then secreted with the bile into the small intestine and eliminated through the intestinal tract in your bowel movements.

Another way to offset excess estrogen is to increase progesterone production by stimulating ovulation. To do this, you need to stimulate the production of the pituitary's luteinizing hormone (LH) so that it is properly balanced with the production of the pituitary's follicle-stimulating hormone (FSH). The imbalances in these hormones in the pituitary upset the normal production of estrogen, progesterone and testosterone by the ovaries and adrenal glands, disrupting the healthy balance between all three of these sex hormones.

Additionally, increasing the production of the different types of neuro-transmitters in the brain—those linked with energy and alertness, as well as those associated with relaxation, calm and sleep—are necessary for healthy menstruation, as they regulate hormone output from the hypothalamus and pituitary, the master hormone-regulating glands in your brain. In turn, these hormones help to stimulate ovulation from your central nervous system.

The end result of my nutritional supplement program is not only relief of your endometriosis symptoms but also healthier and more regular menstrual cycles and less premenstrual and menstrual symptoms. If you are in your forties, it will also help to ensure an easier transition into menopause with fewer symptoms! I have seen this often with my own patients. Let's begin by looking at each step.

Modulate Estrogen Production by Binding to Receptor Sites

As I indicated above, certain plants and nutrients curb estrogen production by binding to the estrogen receptor sites and blocking the enzymes that convert testosterone into estrogen. The key supplements in this process are soy isoflavones, flaxseed oil and lignans and bioflavonoids (mainly from citrus fruit sources). Any of these nutrients can be used by themselves or in combination to help curb estrogen production, depending on your preference.

Soy. Thanks to its weak estrogenic activity, soy reduces the production of more potent estrogens within your body. It does this through its phytoestrogens genistein and daidzein, which belong to the class of chemicals called isoflavones. Soy isoflavones were first discovered during the 1930's, but their potency was not assayed until the 1950's. At that time, genistein was found to be a natural plant estrogen that's 50,000 times weaker than any strong, synthetic form of the hormone.

According to a study from the journal *Cancer*, women who took 40 mg of the soy isoflavone genistein for 12 weeks had a 53 to 55 percent reduction in their estrogen levels. Several similar studies have shown the same results.

To enjoy these types of estrogen-reducing advantages at home, take in 50 to 100 mg of soy isoflavones each day, either through soy foods, isoflavone capsules, or a combination of both. Some women, however, prefer not to use soy because of its side-effects of causing digestive disturbances and should instead use the other options discussed next.

Isoflavone Content of Soy Products

½ cup tofu = 35 mg isoflavones
½ cup tempeh = 35 mg isoflavones
1 cup soy milk = 35–40 mg isoflavones
½ cup edamame (whole soy beans) = 150 mg isoflavones

Flaxseed. Flaxseed is extremely beneficial for the elimination of endometriosis symptoms since it both reduces the production of excess estrogen and also promotes ovulation and progesterone production. It is one of my favorite supplements to help control the symptoms of endometriosis.

Flaxseed is very unusual in its make-up since it contains a double source of plant-based estrogen. Both the oil and the flax lignan (a substance contained within the cellulose-like material that provides structure to plants) contained within the seed have been researched for their estrogenic effect. Once plant lignans are eaten, intestinal bacteria convert them to weakly estrogenic substances that are absorbed into the body.

Lignans inhibit the production of estrogen, as seen in a study conducted at the University of Michigan, and published in the *Journal of Clinical Endocrinology and Metabolism*. Women with normal menstrual cycles ate their usual diet for three cycles and then added 10 grams of flaxseed powder per day to their diet for an additional three cycles.

During the time that the women did not eat flaxseed, there were three cycles when no ovulation occurred. But when flaxseed was included, all of the women in the study ovulated every menstrual cycle. Ovulation, or the release of the egg from the follicle (or casing) in which it is contained at mid-cycle, is necessary for the production of progesterone during the second half of the cycle. Thus, ground flaxseed was found to improve the estrogen-to-progesterone ratio by favoring the production of progesterone within the body. This is very beneficial for estrogen dominant women who suffer from endometriosis as well as PMS, fibroid tumors and other hormone related conditions. In my own clinical practice, I have been thrilled with the benefits of flaxseed in helping to normalize the menstrual cycles in many of my own patients.

Flaxseed also contains fatty acids, from which short lived, hormone-like chemicals called prostaglandins are created. Prostaglandins are another substance that is essential for the process of ovulation to occur. Each of your ovaries contains thousands upon thousands of follicles. These structures contain an ovum (or egg). During each menstrual cycle, one of these follicles becomes the dominant one for that month. At mid-cycle, this dominant follicle will burst or rupture, thereby releasing the egg into the fallopian tube and down into the uterus, where it can then be fertilized and pregnancy can occur. In order for the follicle to rupture and release the ovum, prostaglandins must be present.

To help rebalance estrogen levels and increase ovulation, I recommend taking 1–2 tablespoons of cold-pressed flaxseed oil or 4–6 tablespoons of ground flaxseed daily. Flaxseed oil is sold in opaque containers in the refrigerator section of most health food stores, as it is very sensitive to heat, light, and oxygen. Whole flaxseed is also available, as is pre-ground and capsule form. If you purchase the whole seed, be sure to buy it as a fine meal. Ground flaxseeds are necessary in order to release the beneficial lignans. You can purchase ground flax meal from health food stores or online.

Bioflavonoids. Finally, bioflavonoids can also be used to balance hormone levels, particularly when used in combination with vitamin C. Bioflavonoids are mildly estrogenic antioxidants that are found in the pulp and rind of citrus fruit. They are also anti-estrogenic and help to reduce excessive levels of estrogen in the body. Let me explain this a little further.

Their effect on estrogen production is similar to that of soy isoflavones and flaxseed lignans, as I described earlier. Although bioflavonoids have weak, estrogen-like properties, they have also been shown to interfere with the production of estrogen by competing with estrogen precursors such as androstenedione and testosterone for binding sites on an enzyme called estrogen synthetase. In essence, this blocks the male hormones from being converted into estrogen in the ovaries as well as fatty tissues.

In this way, bioflavonoids work to normalize estrogen balance, bringing excessively high estrogen down to more normal levels. In a related mechanism, bioflavonoids also bind to estrogen receptor sites in the uterus and breasts, blocking your body's own high-octane estrogen from doing damage.

Additionally, studies have shown that bioflavonoids, in combination with vitamin C, also help to reduce heavy menstrual bleeding in transitioning menopausal women, as well as women suffering from bleeding due to fibroid tumors.

Other research indicates the same benefit from flavonoids alone. According to a study from the *Journal of Gynecology and Obstetrics*, flavonoids not only reduce heavy menstrual bleeding, but also ease menstrual cramps. Of the 36 women who took 1,000 mg a day of a flavonoid-based nutritional product for just under 12 months, 70 percent of them enjoyed a 50 percent reduction in their bleeding. In addition, the length of the bleeding time was one-third less. Seventy-five percent of the women also saw a 50 percent reduction in the severity of their menstrual cramps. *I suggest taking 1,000–2,000 mg of citrus bioflavonoids per day along with mineral buffered vitamin C. (Vitamin C is discussed in more detail in the next section). Bioflavonoids are considered very safe and have virtually no side effects.*

Note: In addition to the citrus variety, other specific bioflavonoids such as quercetin and rutin also have anti-estrogen properties. In fact, research studies are finding that quercetin may also help reduce your risk of ovarian cancer. And rutin has been shown to be particularly helpful in strengthening capillaries and reducing heavy menstrual bleeding.

Vitamins for Estrogen Modulation

There are also key vitamins that work to regulate the effects of estrogen on menstrual bleeding and PMS symptoms, as well as promoting healthier menstrual function. These include vitamins C and vitamin E. Vitamin C helps strengthen and fortify blood vessels, thereby reducing heavy menstrual bleeding, particularly when taken with bioflavonoids. According to a study from the *American Journal of Obstetrics and Gynecology*, women who received 600 mg each of both vitamin C and bioflavonoids daily, in divided dosages, for two months experienced less blood loss, as compared to those taking a placebo.

Similarly, a study from *Fertility and Sterility* found vitamin C improved hormone levels and increased fertility in women with luteal phase defect. As I indicated earlier, your menstrual cycle has two phases. The first is the follicular phase, which begins on day one of your period and ends at ovulation. The second luteal phase starts with ovulation and ends on the first day of your period. Estrogen levels rise during the follicular phase, while progesterone levels increase in the luteal phase.

Several factors can prevent adequate progesterone production in the luteal phase, including oxidative stress. That's where vitamin C comes in. A recent study found that women who received 750 mg of vitamin C every day for three months enjoyed increased progesterone levels. Interestingly, those women who did not received vitamin C not only had lower levels of progesterone, but also showed increased levels of estrogen. One reason for this is that vitamin C is necessary to convert essential fatty acids into prostaglandins. Remember, progesterone can only be produced in the ovary during the second half of your menstrual cycle, after ovulation has occurred. *To help lower estrogen levels in your body, I suggest taking 1,000–4,000 mg of mineral-buffered vitamin C per day, in divided doses to prevent diarrhea.*

Another key nutrient is vitamin E. Vitamin E helps to relieve the symptoms of PMS, including menstrual cramps, as well as benign breast disease. Although it is unclear exactly how vitamin E works to relieve PMS symptoms, it is widely believed that either its antioxidant properties or its modulation of prostaglandin production are involved. Research conducted at Johns Hopkins University Medical Center also found that vitamin E helps to reduce discomfort from fibrocystic breasts.

Early research has also shown that vitamin E was useful to reestablish healthy menstrual cycles in young women. Living under the stress of war is often associated with widespread disruption of menstrual cycles. This was true of women living in an internment camp in Manila during World War II. Doctors who treated these women observed that menstruation had stopped abruptly after the first bombing of Manila, before a nutritional deficiency would have been experienced.

These physicians conducted a small study, published in the *Journal of the American Medical Association*, in which women with amenorrhea (a lack of menstruation) were given 20 drops of wheat germ oil (a great source of vitamin E). The doses were taken orally, three times a day, for a period of 10 days, preceding the onset of each woman's expected menstrual flow. Of the 10 women, eight began to experience healthy menstruation.

I suggest taking 400–1,000 IU of natural vitamin E a day, in an oil-based capsule. If you cannot tolerate oil-based products, there is a dry form of vitamin E available. Start with the lower dose and increase by 400 IU every two weeks until the desired effect is achieved.

Note: Vitamin E is considered extremely safe and is commonly used by millions of individuals. However, women with certain medical problems, such as hypertension, insulin-dependent diabetes, and menstrual-bleeding problems, should begin taking vitamin E at lower dosages, starting with 100 IU per day and slowly increasing the dosage. If you have any of these health conditions, check with your doctor before supplementing with vitamin E.

While plant-based nutrients and vitamins all work to reduce your estrogen production, you also need to increase the metabolism and elimination of the hormone. Let's take a look at the best ways to accomplish this.

Estrogen Breakdown

To eliminate excess estrogen from the body, it is also necessary to support the healthy breakdown and elimination of estrogen. This is partly accomplished by our liver. The liver is our main organ of detoxification. When it is working properly, it metabolizes estrogen and converts it into less potent forms of this hormone that have less biological activity. These weaker forms of estrogen are less likely to stimulate the growth of endometriosis implants.

Once the liver has done its job, it secretes estrogen into the bile and from there, the estrogen-laden bile flows into your digestive tract, specifically the small intestine, where it is eliminated through your bowel movements. When this process works smoothly, it helps to keep your estrogen levels balanced and healthy. This entire process is called the enterohepatic circulation of estrogen. Let's look at it now in more detail.

During this process, estrogen circulates in the blood throughout your body and passes through your liver. Your liver then metabolizes it from its more potent forms, estradiol and estrone, to a more chemically inactive and safer form called estriol. When the liver is healthy, this process occurs efficiently. The estrogen metabolites are then secreted into the bile and, from there, into your digestive tract.

There are several substances that help to facilitate this process of detoxifying estrogen. These include the well-known B vitamins, as well as the lesser-known but powerful combination of nutrients including diindolymethane (DIM), calcium-d-glucarate, d-limonene, fiber, and probiotics.

The vitamin B-complex is a group of 11 separate, water-soluble nutrients: B1 (thiamine), B2 (riboflavin), B3 (niacin), B5 (pantothenic acid), B6, B12, biotin, folic acid, para-aminobenzoic acid (PABA), choline and inositol. In addition to regulating mood and restoring energy, B vitamins have been shown to help your liver inactivate estrogen. According to a 1942 study published in *Endocrinology*, a lack of B vitamins negatively affects your liver's ability to detoxify estrogen. Specifically, researchers found that women with several health problems related to excess estrogen levels (heavy menstrual flow, benign breast disease and PMS) who received vitamin B-complex supplements enjoyed relief of their symptoms.

Additionally, like magnesium, B vitamins also help convert essential fatty acids taken in through your diet into inflammation-fighting prostaglandins. This anti-inflammatory effect helps relieve muscle cramps and pelvic discomfort. (I discuss this further on in this chapter).

Finally, a study conducted by Guy Abraham, M.D., at UCLA Medical School found that women who took 500 mg of vitamin B6 for three months enjoyed a reduction in PMS symptoms, including menstrual cramps, pain and weight gain. According to Dr. Abraham, vitamin B6 helped to change the blood levels of both estrogen and progesterone and bring them into balance. This is also very beneficial for the relief of endometriosis.

To help neutralize estrogen and ease symptoms of excess estrogen, I suggest taking 50–100 mg of a vitamin B-complex a day. Be sure it includes 50–100 mg of vitamin B6.

DIM. Diindolylmethane, or DIM, is a plant-compound found in Brassica veggies such as broccoli, bok choy, cauliflower, cabbage, and Brussels sprouts. Researchers have found that this interesting little compound is quite beneficial in promoting estrogen metabolism.

During estrogen metabolism, the most potent form of estrogen (estradiol) is converted into estrone. Estrone then becomes either 2-hydroxyestrone — a "good" estrone metabolite — or 16-alpha-hydroxyestrone — a "bad" estrogen metabolite. The good metabolite (2-hydroxyestrone) is then converted into 2-methoxyestrone and 2-methoxyestrodial.

This is where DIM comes in. Research has shown that when DIM is ingested, it not only encourages its own metabolism, but that of estrogen. While it is not an estrogen or even an estrogen-mimic, its metabolic pathway exactly coincides with the metabolic pathway of estrogen. When these pathways intersect, DIM favorably adjusts the estrogen metabolic pathways by simultaneously increasing the good estrogen metabolites and decreasing the bad 16-alpha-hydroxyestrone.

The research confirms this action. In a study from *Epidemiology*, American researchers took urine samples from healthy postmenopausal women. They then added 10 grams of broccoli a day to the women's diets. After taking another urine sample, researchers found that this dietary change significantly increased the 2-hydroxyestrone to 16-alpha-hydroxyestrone ratio.

In addition to eating more Brassica vegetables like cauliflower and broccoli, I recommend taking 30 mg of DIM a day with meals.

D-Glucarate. Glucuronidation, a detoxification process that occurs in the liver, depends on glucuronic acid, a chemical produced within the body which is similar to calcium d-glucarate, a naturally occurring substance found in many fruits and vegetables.

This process is very important for the elimination of estrogen dominance. As estrogen circulates through the blood, it passes through the liver, where it is bound to glucuronic acid. This binding process inactivates the estrogen, inhibiting it from binding to tissues such as endometriosis implants. It is then secreted into the bile and passed into the intestinal tract, where it is then eliminated from the body via bowel movements.

Unfortunately, certain bacteria in the intestinal tract secrete an enzyme called beta-glucuronidase (B-glucuronidase) which can sabotage the glucuronidation process. B-glucuronidase breaks the newly formed estrogen-glucuronic acid bond apart, which reactivates the estrogen. This free estrogen can then be reabsorbed back into the body, thus elevating the level of estrogen circulating through the body.

Luckily, eating a diet rich in glucarate or using glucarate supplements helps to decrease the level of B-glucuronidase by allowing the bond between glucuronic acid and estrogen to be maintained so the body can rid itself of excess estrogen. This helps to prevent your own level of estrogen from rising to toxic levels.

To reduce the total amount of circulating estrogen, I recommend taking 500 to 1,000 mg of glucarate per day with meals. This supplement is very well tolerated with no toxicity or known drug interactions.

Glucarate-Rich Foods

Apples	Brussels sprouts
Apricots	Cherries
Broccoli	Lettuce

Limonene. Another ally to help lower your total estrogen load is limonene, a compound usually found in citrus fruits, especially lemons and oranges. In addition to supporting glucuronidation, limonene also promotes healthy detoxification. One benefit of limonene is that it has been shown to help prevent the development of estrogen-dependent breast cancer by stimulating detoxification enzymes in the liver.

A study published in *Cancer Research* tested to see if limonene could reduce or regress breast cancer in rats. Researchers fed a limonene-rich diet to rats that had developed breast tumors. They found that the rats that were given this diet had significant tumor shrinkage as compared to the control group. However, when the limonene was discontinued, the tumors reappeared. Additionally, researchers found that limonene inhibited the spread or metastasis of the cancer. ***To help reduce free-floating estrogen in your body, I recommend taking 500–1,000 mg of limonene per day or every other day.***

Note: Women who are allergic to citrus should not take limonene. Additionally, while it appears to be safe and without toxicity, pregnant or nursing women should not take limonene since no research has been performed that specifically examines its effect on fetal development.

Limonene-Rich Foods

Caraway	Oranges
Cherries	Mint
Dill	Tomatoes
Lemons	

Fiber. Once estrogen is broken down and neutralized by your liver, it is secreted into your bile. From there, it enters your small intestines. Within the digestive tract, dietary fiber is a key component to eliminating excess estrogen from your body. Fiber works by binding to estrogen and removing it through bowel movements. According to a study from Tufts University Medical School, vegetarian women excrete two to three times more estrogen in their bowel movements than do other women who eat a diet lower in fiber and higher in fat. This is great news for estrogen dominant women who are trying to reduce the estrogen load in their body.

In addition to regulating estrogen levels, fiber also binds to cholesterol. This helps to keep your bad cholesterol levels in a healthy range.

Plus, fiber is key for preventing constipation, colon cancer and many other intestinal disorders. (More than 85,000 cases of colon cancer are diagnosed each year). Once ingested, fiber undergoes bacterial fermentation in the colon. This process produces butyrate, the main energy source for colonic epithelial cells, which are needed for a healthy, cancer-free colon. This effect was verified in a study published in the *Scandinavian Journal of Gastroenterology*. Researchers followed the health of 20 patients who had undergone surgical treatment for colon cancer. The volunteers were given fiber in the form of psyllium seeds. After one month of supplementation, fecal concentration of butyrate increased by 47 percent.

There are two types of fiber: soluble and insoluble. Soluble fibers (dissolvable in water) are found in fruits, vegetables, nuts and beans. Insoluble fibers (not dissolvable in water) are found in oatmeal, oat bran, sesame seeds, and dried beans. Sadly, the refining process has removed most of the natural fiber from our foods, creating a nation of people grossly lacking in fiber.

To ensure that you are getting adequate amounts of both kinds of fiber (and therefore ensuring the effective elimination of excess estrogen), be sure to eat whole-grain cereals and flours; brown rice; all kinds of bran; fruits such as apricots, prunes, and apples; nuts and seeds; beans, lentils, and peas; and a wide variety of vegetables. Flaxseed is also a great source of dietary fiber. Several of these foods should be included in every meal. Moreover, when you eat apples and potatoes, enjoy them with their skins.

You can further supplement your diet with fibers like oat bran and/or psyllium (1–2 tablespoons per day, mixed with 8–12 ounces of water and swallowed immediately after stirring). You may also try guar gum (which is helpful in regulating your blood sugar level) and pectin (which is derived from apples and grapefruit and can lower the amount of fat that you absorb from your diet). Simply combine ½ teaspoon guar gum and 500 mg of pectin with 8–12 ounces of water. Stir and drink immediately. Use one to three times a day.

Probiotics. Many women with estrogen dominance tend to eat a high-fat, low-fiber diet. High intake of saturated fats, commonly found in foods such as dairy, butter and red meat stimulate the growth of unhealthy, anaerobic bacteria in the intestinal tract. These bacteria chemically change the breakdown products of estrogen into forms that can be reabsorbed back into the body.

These bacteria split estrogen from the binding substances that inactivate it in your liver. This splitting process causes free estrogen to be reformed within your intestinal tract. As this free estrogen is reabsorbed into the circulation, it increases free estrogen levels within the blood.

To suppress the growth of these unhealthy bacteria, I suggest that you not only reduce your intake of saturated fat (which can lead to the problem in the first place), but that you also use probiotic supplements. Probiotics help to recolonize your intestinal tract with healthy bacteria such as L. acidophilus and B. longum. *I recommend taking probiotics that contain at least 1–3 billion live, healthy organisms per day.*

In addition to decreasing the amount of estrogen in your body by reducing its production and increasing its elimination, you can help to offset the hormone by increasing your progesterone levels. To accomplish this, you need to stimulate ovulation at both the central nervous system and ovarian levels.

Balance Excess Estrogen with Progesterone

While estrogen stimulates the growth of endometriosis implants, progesterone helps to limit their growth. The best way I know to increase progesterone production is to stimulate ovulation at mid-cycle. This can be done on two levels, through supporting the health of the central nervous system as well as its production by the ovaries.

Most women are surprised to learn that you can increase progesterone production through the brain or central nervous system. What many people don't realize is that all hormone production begins in the brain. In this section, I discuss two supplements, vitex and maca, that help to balance your hormones through the neurological pathways.

Vitex. Vitex is an herb native to the Mediterranean area. Also known as chaste tree berry, due to its ability to decrease libido, vitex has been used for centuries to ease heavy menstrual bleeding, promote ovulation, and even restore menstruation in women who suffer from amenorrhea.

Vitex works at the hypothalamic and pituitary levels. Specifically, it inhibits the release of FSH, which lowers estrogen production, while also aiding in the production of LH to trigger ovulation, thereby promoting progesterone production.

One study found that vitex helps restore menstruation by increasing progesterone levels. Researchers gave vitex extract to 20 women who had either abnormal or non-existent menstruation. After six months, 15 of the women were available for evaluation. Lab tests revealed that 10 of the 15 women had a return of their menstrual cycles, as well as increased levels of both progesterone and LH. Their FSH levels either remained consistent or decreased slightly.

A similar study found that eight women with abnormally low progesterone levels who were given vitex every day for three months also enjoyed increased progesterone levels. In fact, two of the women became pregnant!

Vitex has also been shown to hinder the release of prolactin, a hormone closely related to human growth hormone, which plays a critical role in lactation. If there is too much prolactin in your system, secretion of LH is disturbed, which in turn can disrupt ovulation, and therefore progesterone production.

Several studies have proven vitex's ability to reduce prolactin levels. One double-blind, placebo-controlled study examined 52 women with luteal phase problems due to increased prolactin levels. They were given 20 mg of vitex a day for three months. At the end of the treatment period, prolactin levels had been significantly reduced.

Similarly, a German study looked at 13 women between the ages of 15 and 48 years, all of whom suffered from menstrual dysfunction. Lab tests showed that all the women had abnormally high prolactin levels. After taking vitex for three months, all the women had "continuous and significant" decreases in their prolactin levels.

A study from *Experimental and Clinical Endocrinology* suggests that vitex works to decrease prolactin by binding to dopamine receptors, which in turn thwart the secretion of prolactin. Interestingly, the researchers found that while prolactin secretion was inhibited, gonadotropin secretion (which leads to FSH and LH secretion) remained unaffected.

Research from several German peer-reviewed publications confirms this finding. For example, the *International Journal of Gynecology & Obstetrics*, and Hormone and Metabolic Research have both found that vitex appears to block prolactin secretion by binding to dopamine receptors. However, much research still needs to be done in this area.

To increase progesterone levels and decrease prolactin, I suggest taking 140–275 mg of a standardized extract of vitex (chaste tree berry) every day. Chaste tree berry works slowly, so it may take three or four months before you start to see its full benefit.

Maca. Maca is referred to as either Lepidium peruvianum or Lepidium meyenii. It is one of the most traditionally used and valued Peruvian herbs, due in large part to its rich nutrient concentration. This malty, butter-scotch-flavored root contains a number of minerals, vitamins, fatty acids, plant sterols, amino acids, and alkaloids, among other phyto-nutrients. In terms of minerals, calcium makes up 10 percent of maca's mineral content. Magnesium, phosphorus, and potassium are also present in significant amounts. Maca also contains a number of vitamins and amino acids, including B1, B2, B12, vitamin C, vitamin E, and quercetin, as well as arginine, lysine, tryptophan, tyrosine, and phenylalanine.

German and American researchers begin studying Peruvian botanicals in the 1960's and 1980's. They quickly discovered that maca has many health benefits, including relieving menopausal symptoms; stimulating and regulating the endocrine system (adrenals, thyroid, ovaries, and testes); increasing energy, stamina, and endurance; regulating and normalizing menstrual cycles; and balancing hormone levels.

Maca appears to act as a central nervous system stimulant, at the level of the hypothalamus and pituitary gland. It works to stimulate hormone production, which is a critical part of regulating a woman's physiology. It also operates as an adaptogenic herb to help regulate hormones produced by the endocrine glands. It does this by stimulating your ovaries and adrenals to produce the hormones you need; in the levels you need them.

This was shown in a study published in the *Journal of Veterinary Medical Science*. Researchers tested the effects of maca on mouse sex hormones. They found that while progesterone and testosterone levels increased significantly in the mice that received the maca, their estradiol levels were not increased. In other words, the maca helped to raise the levels of progesterone and testosterone to offset the blood levels of estradiol in the mice. This is exciting news for women suffering from estrogen dominance.

A traditional dosage of maca is 2–10 grams a day. However, dosages are unique to each woman, so you will need to determine which dosage works for you. There have been no acute toxic effects of maca, even at very high doses. In fact, many Peruvians eat it every day!

Note: If you are sensitive or allergic to herbs, you may want to use maca cautiously. In any event, I suggest starting with the low end of the recommended dosage, as too much can cause increased hot flashes, breast tenderness, or headaches. It is also recommended that you avoid maca if you have a hormone-related cancer (due to lack of formal studies), liver disease, if you are pregnant or nursing, or if you are currently taking conventional HRT.

While stimulating progesterone production originates in your central nervous system, you also need to support your ovaries and adrenals, which also support progesterone production. Here's a look at the three key nutrients that support its production in the ovaries.

Ovarian Progesterone Production

Progesterone (as well as estrogen and testosterone) are produced by your ovaries and adrenals. It is very important to keep these essential endocrine glands functioning at their optimal level for healthy progesterone levels. To do this, I highly recommend using the following key nutrients: lutein, beta-carotene, and essential fatty acids. I also discuss the use of natural bioidentical progesterone therapy.

Lutein. Lutein is a carotenoid with powerful antioxidant properties and cell protective benefits. It is a beautiful yellow colored phytonutrient found in flowers like marigolds, fruits and vegetables. Many women are aware of its benefits for healthy vision, but lutein is just as important for supporting a healthy balance between your estrogen and progesterone levels.

Lutein is found abundantly in the ovaries and is present in very high concentrations in the corpus luteum, or yellow body, of the ovary. The corpus luteum produces your progesterone and estrogen during the second half of the menstrual cycle. (In contrast, only estrogen is formed during the first half of the menstrual cycle).

During ovulation, the follicle (or casing) that contains the egg is ruptured. This allows the egg or ovum to be expelled from the ovary and migrate to the uterus where it can undergo fertilization, which results in pregnancy, or else breaks down and leaves the body with menstruation. Once the egg is released from the follicle, the follicle is then converted into a new structure called the corpus luteum. Lutein is abundant in the corpus luteum and provides it with its distinctive yellow color.

As already mentioned, he purpose of the corpus luteum is to switch from the estrogen production, which predominates during the first half of the menstrual cycle (days one to 14) to the production of progesterone and estrogen during the second half of your cycle (days 15 to 28). This is called the luteinizing process. During this time, lutein begins to accumulate on these key cells, and the effectiveness of the luteinizing process may be due, in part, to the amount of lutein found there.

Great food sources of lutein include my favorite greens like spinach, kale, collard greens, turnip greens, as well as romaine lettuce, broccoli, Brussels sprouts, various squashes and green peas. Lutein is also abundantly present in egg yolk, corn, kiwi fruit, grapes and orange juice.

To ensure that you have adequate lutein levels to support normal development of the corpus luteum, I suggest supplementing with 6–12 mg of lutein a day.

Beta-Carotene. Beta-carotene is the plant-based, water-soluble precursor to vitamin A. Like lutein, beta-carotene is abundant in the ovaries, and is found in very high concentrations in the corpus luteum and the adrenal glands—both of which produce progesterone. Some research even suggests that a proper balance between carotene and the retinal form of vitamin A is necessary for proper luteal function.

Researchers have been aware of the reproductive benefits of beta-carotene for more than a century. For example, cows whose diets were deficient in beta-carotene experienced delayed ovulation, decreased progesterone levels, and an increased prevalence of ovarian cysts, as well as cystic mastitis (breast cysts). Both conditions are typically found in women who are progesterone deficient.

Research studies have also found carotenoids such as beta-carotene, as well as vitamin A, to be useful in treating conditions related to estrogen dominance, including ovarian cancer, heavy menstrual bleeding, and benign breast disease. A study from the *International Journal of Cancer* found that high carotenoid intake decreased a woman's risk for ovarian cancer. In fact, beta-carotene rich carrots were among the foods most strongly associated with decreased risk.

Studies have also determined that vitamin A helps prevent heavy menstrual bleeding. Researchers tested the blood levels of 71 women suffering with excessive bleeding. They found that all the women had lower than normal levels of vitamin A. After taking vitamin A supplements for just two weeks, 90 percent of them returned to normal menstruation levels.

Finally, a study from *Preventative Medicine* found that high doses of vitamin A can help reverse one form of benign breast disease. Researchers gave 150,000 IU of vitamin A to 12 women with fibrocystic breasts. After three months, more than half the women reported complete or partial remission of the cysts. While I would never suggest that women take this high a dose of vitamin A for fear of toxicity, I believe that beta-carotene would have a similar effect.

Foods rich in beta-carotene include carrots, pumpkins, sweet red peppers, papayas, apricots, kale, collards and dandelion greens.

To ensure that you have adequate amounts of beta-carotene in your system, I suggest taking 10,000–25,000 IU a day.

Essential Fatty Acids. Essential fatty acids (EFAs) are health-promoting nutrients that your body needs to perform a whole range of functions. There are two main groups of EFAs: the omega-3 family and the omega-6 family. The most common are linoleic acid (omega-6) and the omega-3 fatty acids alpha-linolenic acid, eicosapentaenoic acid (EPA) and docosahexaenoic acid (DHA). Both essential fatty acid families must be derived from dietary sources because they cannot be produced within the body.

Your body converts EFAs into series-1 and 3 prostaglandins, potent hormone-like substances with a wide range of benefits that are essential for good reproductive health. Among other things, these prostaglandins help to promote more frequent ovulation at mid-cycle. Since prostaglandins are necessary for the rupture of the follicle, which allows the egg to be extruded from the ovary at mid-cycle, this is a critical step for progesterone production to occur during the second half of the cycle.

The two best sources of EFAs are flaxseed and fish oil. I discussed flaxseed earlier in this chapter in relationship to its benefits in reducing estrogen dominance. Plus, flax has been proven to support progesterone production. Researchers at the University of Michigan tested women with normal menstrual cycles. During three cycles, the women ate as they normally would. They then added 10 grams of ground flaxseed per day to their diet for an additional three cycles. The women who ate flaxseed had more ovulatory cycles than the women who did not. In addition, ground flaxseed was found to improve the estrogen-to-progesterone ratio, favoring the levels of progesterone within the body. The researchers felt that this was due to the lignans contained in the flaxseed, although I feel strongly that the flaxseed oil was also very beneficial in this regard, as it is also converted into prostaglandins, which are necessary for ovulation to occur. . In the case of flaxseed, both the oil and the ground meal are rich in EFAs. *To promote progesterone production, I suggest taking 1–2 tablespoons of flaxseed oil or 4–6 tablespoons of ground flaxseed per day.*

If you do not like flaxseed or cannot tolerate it, you may prefer to get your EFAs through fish oil. In addition to promoting progesterone production and helping to regulate the menstrual cycle, fish oil is extremely beneficial for easing menstrual cramps, endometriosis, and breast cysts due to its anti-inflammatory benefits.

EFAs derived from fish oil are effective for a wide variety of estrogen dominant-related conditions, but they are most commonly heralded for their effectiveness in easing menstrual cramps. This is very beneficial if you are suffering from pain and cramping due to endometriosis. Specifically, a study from the *American Journal of Obstetrics and Gynecology* looked at 42 girls between the ages of 15 and 18 years, all of whom had experienced significant menstrual pain during their periods. Those girls who took 1,080 mg of EPA and 720 mg of DHA every day for two months enjoyed a significant decrease in their pain due to menstrual cramps. No change was observed in the placebo group. Additionally, the amount of painkillers the girls took during their menstrual periods decreased by more than 50 percent during the fish oil treatment as compared to the placebo treatment.

If fish oil is your preference, I suggest taking between 2000- 3000 mg DHA and EPA combined every day. Vegetarians can use algae (seaweed) sources of DHA and EPA.

Iron. Women who suffer from heavy menstrual bleeding due to endometriosis tend to be iron deficient. In fact, some medical studies have found that inadequate iron intake may even cause excessive bleeding. Women who suffer from heavy menstrual bleeding should have their red blood count checked to see if they need supplemental iron in addition to a high-iron-content diet. Heme iron, the iron from meat sources like liver, is much better absorbed and assimilated than non-heme iron, the iron from vegetarian sources. To be absorbed properly, non-heme iron must be taken with at least 75 milligrams of vitamin C.

Iron deficiency is the main cause of anemia due to heavy menstrual flow. Iron is an essential component of red blood cells, combining with protein and copper to make hemoglobin, the pigment of the red blood cells. Iron deficiency is common during all phases of a woman's life and is a frequent cause of fatigue and low-energy states. Good food sources of iron include liver, blackstrap molasses, beans and peas, seeds and nuts, and certain fruits and vegetables.

Natural Progesterone. Natural progesterone is produced in the laboratory from diosgenin, the active component of soybeans or the Mexican wild yam, as are pregnenolone and DHEA. While synthesized in the laboratory, it has the same chemical structure and range of activity as the progesterone made by the body. Since progesterone has a growth limiting and maturational effect on tissues like the uterus, the lining of the uterus, and breasts, its use counters the effect that unopposed estrogen has on and endometrial implants during perimenopause. It is at this time that these conditions can accelerate greatly.

For women in the late perimenopause who are not ovulating regularly, and therefore producing progesterone less frequently, replacement therapy with natural progesterone may be beneficial in slowing the progression of endometriosis.

Natural progesterone is available in an oral micronized form through a doctor's prescription or over-the-counter as a skin cream. The oral micronized form protects progesterone from being destroyed by the stomach and digestive enzymes. This allows it to be absorbed and utilized by the body. Dosages are 100 to 200 mg. daily but can vary in either direction and should be used for 10 to 12 days per month. Progesterone skin cream can be bought in natural food stores and should contain at least 450 mg per ounce. Rub ¼ to ½ teaspoon directly into the skin twice a day for 10 to 12 days per month. Blood or saliva testing of progesterone levels will help to determine if it is in the therapeutic range.

Anti-Inflammatory Nutritional Supplements

The second part of my nutritional supplement program involves the use of anti-inflammatory substances that help to reduce the pain, cramps and even the spread of the endometriosis implants. I have found these nutrients to be very useful in controlling uncomfortable endometriosis symptoms.

Anti-Inflammatory Digestive Enzymes. Several digestive enzymes can be quite useful in relieving the pain associated with endometriosis. They can also help to reduce scarring and inflammation of the implants that occur with this disease. These enzymes include: bromelain, a digestive enzyme extracted from the stem of the pineapple (500 to 1000 mg. four times a day taken apart from meals); papain, an enzyme derived from papaya (200 to 300 mg. four times a day apart from meals); and pancreatin, which is derived from the pancreas of animals (one to two 300 to 500 mg. four times a day apart from meals). Other useful anti-inflammatories include quercitin, a potent antioxidant (300 to 600 mg. per day), and MSM (250 to 750 mg. per day).

Nattokinase. This substance is an enzyme derived from natto, a food made from fermented soybeans and primarily eaten in Japan. Natto is a traditional Japanese food with a long history of use. The benefits of nattokinase for endometriosis are thought to be due to its ability to dissolve fibrin that forms the mesh structure in blood clots. It is also thought to break down the adhesions, or scar tissue, that are commonly associated with endometriosis and form from the inflammation and recurrent bleeding that is seen with this condition.

Nattokinase should be used with caution by women who are on anti-clotting drugs like Coumadin since it can increase the risk of bleeding or hemorrhage. The same cautions apply to drugs that cause thinning of the blood like aspirin and ibuprofen. The therapeutic dosage is 2000 fibrin degradation units (FU) of activity per serving.

Turmeric (curcumin). Turmeric has been used for thousands of years in Indian cooking and in India's traditional Ayurvedic medicine. The turmeric plant, grown from India to Indonesia, is related to ginger and has pulpy, orange, tuberous roots that grow to about two feet in length. It is an indispensable part of the mixture of spices known as curry powder. The medicinally active compound in turmeric is curcumin, the rich orange-yellow pigment that gives turmeric its characteristic orange-yellow color.

For thousands of years, curcumin has been used in both Chinese and Indian systems of medicine as an anti-inflammatory agent and for the treatment of numerous health conditions. Modern research corroborates its use as an anti-inflammatory. Studies have noted that an added benefit of curcumin is that it does not normally cause side effects, providing a safe alternative to these powerful anti-inflammatory drugs, which can cause gastric irritation and even peptic ulcers in susceptible people.

Curcumin's therapeutic benefits occur through several mechanisms. Curcumin reduces inflammation by inhibiting leukotriene formation and platelet aggregation. It also promotes the breakup of blood clots and inhibits the inflammatory response to various stimuli. There is some indication that curcumin has an indirect effect on reducing inflammation through the adrenal gland or its hormones.

The most likely explanation is that it increases the effectiveness of the body's own cortisone, one of the body's major anti-inflammatory hormones. Curcumin may do this by sensitizing or priming cortisone receptor sites, thereby potentiating cortisone's action. It may also act by increasing the half-life of cortisone through reducing its breakdown by the liver. While the long-term use of prescription cortisone has been associated with serious side effects, including adrenal atrophy, osteoporosis, and diabetes mellitus, curcumin has been found to be as effective as cortisone with no toxicity.

Curcumin also appears to have benefits in reducing the inflammation of endometriosis, both through use in the clinical treatment of endometriosis as well as in animal studies. One study reported in the Indian Journal of Biochemistry and Biophysics found that curcumin had strong anti-endometriosis benefits in an animal model.

The recommended dosage for curcumin as an anti-inflammatory agent is 400 to 600 mg three times a day. It is often formulated with an equal amount of bromelain to enhance absorption. This combination is best taken on an empty stomach, twenty minutes before meals or between meals. Toxicity reactions have not been reported at standard dosage levels.

Anti-Inflammatory Essential Fatty Acids. I discussed fatty acids earlier in the context of their crucial role of helping to promote healthy ovulation and hormonal balance. As mentioned earlier in this chapter, they help to promote more frequent ovulation at mid-cycle, and therefore more menstrual cycles where progesterone is produced. Progesterone helps to limit the growth of endometrial implants. Now let's look at their role in controlling inflammation.

Another great benefit of essential fatty acids is that they are the raw materials from which the beneficial hormone-like chemicals called prostaglandins are made. Prostaglandins are potent anti-inflammatory chemicals that are very beneficial in reducing and preventing inflammation in endometriosis.

By helping to limit inflammation within the endometrial implants (as well as having muscle and blood vessel relaxant effects on tissues like the uterus and fallopian tubes), painful pelvic symptoms can be greatly reduced.

Beneficial prostaglandins are produced from linoleic acid (omega-6 family) and alpha-linolenic acid (omega-3 family). They are derived primarily from raw seeds, nuts, and green leafy vegetables. Other beneficial anti-inflammatory omega-3 fatty acids eicosapentaenoic acid (EPA) and docosahexaenoic acid (DHA) are found in certain fish such as salmon, tuna, eel, mackerel, and trout. Flaxseed oil is the best source of both linoleic and alpha-linolenic acid. Unlike the unhealthy saturated fats, these fats cannot be made by the body and must be supplied daily in our diets, through either food or supplements.

Even when these fatty acids are supplied in the diet, some women lack the ability to convert them efficiently to the muscle-relaxant prostaglandin series-1 prostaglandins. This is particularly true with linoleic acid, which must be converted to a chemical called gamma-linolenic acid (GLA) on its way to becoming the series-1 prostaglandin called E1.

Linoleic acid (omega-6 family) by itself can be found in seeds and seed oils. Good sources include safflower oil, sunflower oil, corn oil, and sesame seed oil. Many women prefer to use raw fresh sesame seeds and sunflower seeds to obtain the oils. Most of us take in abundant amounts of these oils in our diet and they do not need to be further supplemented. The difficulty lies in the conversion of linoleic acid to GLA, followed by the chemical steps leading to the creation of the beneficial prostaglandins. This requires the presence of magnesium, vitamin B6, zinc, vitamin C, and niacin. Women who are deficient in these nutrients can't make the chemical conversions effectively.

In addition, women who eat a high-cholesterol diet, eat processed oils like mayonnaise, use a great deal of alcohol, or are diabetic may have difficulty converting fatty acids to series-1 prostaglandins. Other factors that impede prostaglandin production include emotional stress, allergies, and eczema. In women with these risk factors, less than one percent of linoleic acid may be converted to GLA. The rest of the fatty acids can be used as an energy source, but they will not be able to play a role in relieving menstrual pain, cramp symptoms, and inflammation due to endometriosis.

It is important to note that not all prostaglandins are beneficial. The series-2 prostaglandins derived from the arachidonic acid found in red meat and dairy products can worsen the inflammation of endometriosis. Red meat, dairy products and other sources of saturated fat should be totally eliminated or significantly limited in the diet of women with endometriosis related inflammation.

A number of interesting studies have been done on essential fatty acids as a treatment for PMS. This is particularly relevant for women suffering from endometriosis because PMS often accompanies these problems. Women with PMS often have the congestive type of menstrual cramps with bloating, weight gain, and dull aching pain in the pelvic region. Clinical studies have shown that the use of essential fatty acids can reduce most PMS symptoms by as much as 70 percent. Evening primrose oil, borage oil, and black currant oil are the most common supplemental sources of essential fatty acids for the treatment of menstrual cramps and PMS. All three oils contain high levels of GLA, allowing women to circumvent the difficult conversion process of linoleic acid to GLA.

The best food sources of essential fatty acids are raw flaxseed oil and pumpkin seed oil, which contain high levels of both linoleic acid and alpha-linolenic acid, in combination. Both the seeds and their pressed oils should be used absolutely fresh and unspoiled. Because these oils become rancid very easily when exposed to light and air (oxygen), they need to be packed in opaque containers and kept in the refrigerator. They can also be taken in capsule form.

Fresh flaxseed oil—golden, rich, and delicious—is my special favorite. Good quality flaxseed oil is available in health food stores. Flaxseed oil is extremely high in linoleic and alpha-linolenic acid, which comprises approximately 75 percent of its total content. While it can be added to foods as a butter substitute, flaxseed oil must not be heated. I use it at home on popcorn and steamed vegetables. Use 1 to 2 tablespoons per day of the flaxseed oil or 2 to 6 tablespoons of ground flax meal.

Pumpkin seed oil has a deep green color and spicy flavor. A good source of this oil is fresh raw pumpkin seeds. The raw seeds can be purchased from a health food store and should be kept refrigerated because they are highly perishable. Both flaxseed oil and pumpkin seed oil can also be taken in capsule form.

Omega-3 fatty acids are also found in abundance in fish oils. The best sources are cold-water, high-fat fish such as salmon, tuna, rainbow trout, mackerel, and eel. Fish can be used in your diet once or twice a week but more frequent use of fish should be limited because of the high levels of mercury found in many fish. Instead, I recommend using mercury free fish oil capsules as a daily supplement. You should use fish oil supplements which contain 2000-3000 mg of eicosapentaenoic acid (EPA) and docosa-hexaenoic acid (DHA), the anti-inflammatory omega-3 fatty acids which are found in fish. Vegetarians can use algae (seaweed) supplements of DHA and EPA

The average healthy adult requires only four teaspoons per day of the essential oils, although women with menstrual cramps and pain due to endometriosis may need several tablespoons per day, especially of the anti-inflammatory omega-3 fatty acids like fish oil and flaxseed oil. If you use whole flaxseed, remember that the seeds are 30 percent oil by content, so you need two-thirds as much whole seed intake as oil for the same amount of fatty acids. For optimal results use these oils along with vitamin E, which helps to prevent rancidity of the oils.

Minerals That Reduce Pain and Cramping Due to Inflammation

Certain minerals are very useful in reducing the pain and cramping of endometriosis due to inflammation. These include calcium, magnesium and potassium. I discuss them in detail in this section.

Calcium. This important mineral helps to prevent menstrual pain and cramps by maintaining normal muscle tone. Because cramps are common with endometriosis, calcium intake is important to help prevent further muscular irritability. When taken before bed at night, calcium is effective in helping to combat insomnia due to menstrual discomfort. Muscles that are calcium deficient tend to be hyperactive and more likely to cramp. Since the uterus is made up of muscle, it is susceptible to calcium deficiency.

Calcium is also quite successful in alleviating the PMS-related symptoms that often accompanies endometriosis. A study from the *American Journal of Obstetrics and Gynecology* looked at the effect calcium had on reducing PMS symptoms such as mood swings, bloating, food cravings, and menstrual cramps. They divided 466 women into two groups. The first received 1,200 mg of calcium a day and the other received a placebo over the course of three months. By the end of the third month, those women taking the calcium saw a 48 percent decrease in their PMS symptoms.

Besides promoting normal muscle tone and activity, calcium is a major structural component of bone. Unfortunately, calcium deficiency is common in our society. The recommended daily allowance (RDA) for calcium in menstruating women is 800 milligrams per day and rises to as much as 1500 milligrams per day in postmenopausal women. The typical American diet supplies only about 450 to 550 milligrams per day. No wonder so many American women are at risk for problems like menstrual cramps and osteoporosis. Good food sources of calcium include green leafy vegetables, beans and peas, seeds and nuts, blackstrap molasses, and seafood. *To enjoy relief from your PMS symptoms caused by excess estrogen and take in adequate levels of calcium, I recommend taking 800-1000 mg of calcium carbonate a day.*

Magnesium. Magnesium has an important effect on the neuromuscular system in reducing menstrual cramps and pain. A deficiency of magnesium increases muscular hyperactivity and can worsen menstrual pain that is already severe due to endometriosis. Magnesium optimizes the amount of usable calcium in your system by increasing calcium absorption. Conversely, calcium can interfere with magnesium absorption.

Magnesium significantly mitigates endometriosis and menstrual pain as well as PMS symptoms that often accompany endometriosis. PMS symptoms, including mood changes, pain, inflammation, and breast cysts are reduced by adequate magnesium intake. According to a study conducted at the University of Reading in England and published in the *Journal of Women's Health and Gender-Based Medicine*, magnesium eased water retention and bloating in women suffering from PMS. A follow-up study also suggested that the same amount of magnesium, taken with 50 mg of vitamin B6, eased PMS-related anxiety.

Like vitamin C, magnesium and vitamin B6 are also critical to convert essential fatty acids (like those found in flaxseed, cold-water fish, walnuts, soy, and green leafy vegetables) into beneficial, inflammation-fighting prostaglandins. Like calcium, magnesium is an important structural component of healthy bone tissue, necessary for the prevention of osteoporosis.

It is usually recommended that the diet include half as much magnesium as calcium, or approximately 400 milligrams per day. Most women get only one-third to one-half of this amount in their daily diet, putting them at high risk for menstrual cramping and pain. *I suggest taking 500-800 mg of magnesium with 50–100 of vitamin B6 per day.*

Potassium. Potassium is the third mineral, along with calcium and magnesium, which helps reduce cramps by regulating muscle contraction. Thus, adequate levels of potassium in the body are necessary to prevent worsening of menstrual pain and cramps. Women deficient in potassium may suffer from premenstrual uterine cramping, leg cramps, and even irregular heartbeats. Potassium also plays a role in the maintenance of fluid balance and energy levels. Women low in potassium are more prone to PMS-related bloating, fatigue, and weakness. Women suffering from endometriosis-related diarrhea may lose significant amounts of potassium through watery bowel movements.

For women suffering from these symptoms, the use of a potassium supplement may be helpful. The most common dose avail-able is a 99-milligram tablet or capsule. I generally recommend taking one to three per day for up to one week premenstrually. Potassium, however, must be used cautiously. It should be avoided by women with kidney or cardiovascular disease, because a high level of potassium can cause an irregular heartbeat in women with these problems. Also, potassium can be irritating to the intestinal tract, so it should be taken with meals.

Nutritional Supplements for Women with Endometriosis

Good dietary habits are crucial for control of your endometriosis symptoms. But for many women, the use of nutritional supplements is important in order to achieve high levels of the essential nutrients needed to heal endometriosis. On the following pages is a sample of the vitamins and minerals as well as their dosages that can be used as a foundation for your program. You can also add the other nutrients like flaxseed oil, fish oil and digestive enzymes that I have discussed in this chapter to fill out your program.

You may find it easier to implement your program if you start with one of the better quality multi-nutrient products for women that are available in health food stores and through the Internet and then add the remaining essential nutrients. Remember that all women differ somewhat in their nutritional needs. If you do take the recommended vitamin or herbal supplements, I usually advise that you start with one-fourth to one-half the dose recommended in this book and work your way up slowly to the higher dosage, if needed. You may find that you do best with slightly more or less of certain ingredients.

I recommend that patients take their supplements with meals or at least a snack. Very rarely, a woman will have a digestive reaction to supplements, such as nausea or indigestion. If this happens, stop all supplements; then resume using them, adding one at a time, until you find the offending nutrient. Eliminate from your program any nutrient to which you have a reaction. If you have any specific questions, ask a health-care professional who is knowledgeable about nutrition.

Optimal Nutritional Supplementation for Endometriosis

Vitamins and Minerals	Maximum Daily Dose
Vitamin A	5000 I.U.
Beta-carotene (provitamin A)	10,000 – 25,000 I.U.
Vitamin B-complex	
B1 (thiamine)	25 - 100 mg
B2 (riboflavin)	25 - 100 mg
B3 (niacinamide)	25 - 100 mg
B5 (pantothenic acid)	25 - 100 mg
B6 (pyridoxine)	50 – 100 mg
B12 (cyanocobalamin)	100 – 750 mcg
Folic acid	400 – 800 mcg
Biotin	200 - 500 mcg
Choline	25 - 100 mg
Inositol	25 - 100 mg
PABA	25 - 100 mg
Vitamin C (as mineral ascorbates)	1000-4000 mg
Vitamin D	1000 I.U.
Bioflavonoids	1000-2000 mg
Rutin	200 mg
Vitamin E (d-alpha tocopherol acetate)	800-1600 I.U.
Calcium	1000 - 1200 mg
Magnesium	500 - 600 mg
Potassium	100 mg
Iron	18 mg
Zinc	15 mg
Iodine	150 mcg
Manganese	5 mg
Copper	2 mg
Selenium	200 mcg
Chromium	100 – 200 mcg
Boron	3 mg

Summary Chart For Nutritional Supplements

I want to end this section by summarizing the steps that you can take to help eliminate your endometriosis symptoms through the use of nutritional supplements. These include:

1. Decreasing estrogen production with soy, bioflavonoids and flaxseed.

2. Regulating the effect of estrogen on menstrual function and menstrual bleeding with vitamin C and vitamin E

3. Assisting the breakdown of estrogen in the liver, gallbladder, and intestines with B vitamins, DIM, glucarate and limonene.

4. Enhancing the elimination of excess estrogen with fiber and probiotics.

5. Stimulating ovulation and progesterone production at both the level of the brain and the ovary with vitex, maca, lutein, beta-carotene, essential fatty acids, natural progesterone and additionally iron for bleeding.

6. Reducing inflammation with pancreatin, bromelain, papain, quercitin, MSM, nattokinase, turmeric, essential fatty acids, calcium, magnesium and potassium.

Food Sources of Vitamin A

Vegetables	Fruits	Meat, poultry, seafood
Carrots	Apricots	Crab
Carrot juice	Avocado	Halibut
Collard greens	Cantaloupe	Liver — all types
Dandelion greens	Mangoes	Mackerel
Green onions	Papaya	Salmon
Kale	Peaches	Swordfish
Parsley	Persimmons	
Spinach		
Sweet potatoes		
Turnip greens		
Winter squash		

Food Sources of Vitamin B-Complex (including folic acid)

Vegetables	Legumes	Grains
Alfalfa	Garbanzo beans	Barley
Artichoke	Lentils	Bran
Asparagus	Lima beans	Brown rice
Beets	Pinto beans	Corn Millet
Broccoli	Soybeans	Rice bran
Brussels sprouts		Wheat
Cabbage	*Meat, poultry, seafood*	Wheat germ
Cauliflower	Egg yolks*	
Green beans	Liver*	*Sweeteners*
Kale		Blackstrap molasses
Leeks		
Onions		
Peas		
Romaine lettuce		

Eggs and meat should be from organic, range-free stock fed on pesticide-free food.

Food Sources of Vitamin B6

Grains
Brown rice
Buckwheat flour
Rice bran
Rye flour
Wheat germ
Whole wheat flour

Vegetables
Asparagus
Beet greens
Broccoli
Brussels sprouts
Cauliflower
Green peas
Leeks
Sweet potatoes

Meat, poultry, seafood
Chicken
Salmon
Shrimp
Tuna

Nuts and seeds
Sunflower seeds

Food Sources of Vitamin C

Fruits
Blackberries
Black currants
Cantaloupe
Elderberries
Grapefruit
Grapefruit juice
Guavas
Kiwi fruit
Mangoes
Oranges
Orange juice
Pineapple
Raspberries
Strawberries
Tangerines
Tomatoes

Vegetables and legumes
Asparagus
Black-eyed peas
Broccoli
Brussels sprouts
Cabbage
Cauliflower
Collards
Green onions
Green peas
Kale
Kohlrabi
Parsley
Potatoes
Rutabagas
Sweet pepper
Sweet potatoes
Turnips

Meat, poultry, seafood
Liver — all types
Pheasant
Quail
Salmon

Food Sources of Vitamin E

Vegetables
Asparagus
Cucumber
Green peas
Kale

Nuts and seeds
Almonds
Brazil nuts
Hazelnuts
Peanuts

Meats, poultry, seafood
Haddock
Herring
Mackerel
Lamb
Liver—all types

Oils
Corn
Peanut
Safflower
Sesame
Soybean
Wheat germ

Grains
Brown rice
Millet

Fruits
Mangoes

Food Sources of Essential Fatty Acids

Oils
Flax
Pumpkin
Soybean
Walnut
Safflower

Sunflower
Grape
Corn
Wheat germ
Sesame

Food Sources of Calcium

Vegetables and legumes
Artichoke
Black beans
Black-eyed peas
Beet greens
Broccoli
Brussels sprouts
Cabbage
Collards
Eggplant
Garbanzo beans
Green beans
Green onions
Kale
Kidney beans
Leeks
Lentils
Parsley
Parsnips
Pinto beans
Rutabagas
Soybeans
Spinach
Turnips
Watercress

Meat, poultry, seafood
Abalone
Beef
Bluefish
Carp
Crab
Haddock
Herring
Lamb
Lobster
Oysters
Perch
Salmon
Shrimp
Venison

Fruits
Blackberries
Black currants
Boysenberries
Oranges
Pineapple juice
Prunes
Raisins
Rhubarb
Tangerine juice

Grains
Bran
Brown rice
Bulgar wheat
Millet

Food Sources of Iron

Grains
Bran cereal (All-Bran)
Bran muffin
Millet, dry
Oat flakes
Pasta, whole wheat
Pumpernickel bread
Wheat germ

Legumes
Black beans
Black-eyed peas
Garbanzo beans
Kidney beans
Lentils
Lima beans
Pinto beans
Soybeans
Split peas
Tofu

Vegetables
Beets
Beet greens
Broccoli
Brussels sprouts
Corn
Dandelion greens
Green beans
Kale
Leeks
Spinach
Sweet potatoes
Swiss chard

Fruits
Apple juice
Avocado
Blackberries
Dates, dried
Figs
Prunes, dried
Prune juice
Raisins

Meat, poultry, seafood
Beef liver
Calf's liver
Chicken liver
Clams
Oysters
Sardines
Scallops
Trout

Nuts and seeds
Almonds
Pecans
Pistachios
Sesame butter
Sesame seeds
Sunflower seeds

Food Sources of Magnesium

Vegetables and legumes
Artichoke
Black-eyed peas
Carrot juice
Corn
Green peas
Leeks
Lima beans
Okra
Parsnips
Potatoes
Soybean sprouts
Spinach
Squash
Yams
Turkey

Grains
Millet
Brown rice
Wild rice

Meat, poultry, seafood
Beef
Carp
Chicken
Clams
Cod
Crab
Duck
Haddock
Herring
Lamb
Mackerel
Oysters
Salmon
Shrimp
Snapper

Nuts and seeds
Almonds
Brazil nuts
Hazelnuts
Peanuts
Pistachios
Pumpkin seeds
Sesame seeds
Walnuts

Fruits
Avocado
Banana
Grapefruit juice
Pineapple juice
Raisins
Papaya
Prunes

Food Sources of Potassium

Vegetables and legumes	Meat, poultry, seafood	Nuts and seeds
Artichoke	Bass	Almonds
Asparagus	Beef	Brazil nuts
Black-eyed peas	Carp	Chestnuts
Beets	Catfish	Hazelnuts
Brussels sprouts	Chicken	Macadamia nuts
Carrot juice	Cod	Peanuts
Cauliflower	Duck	Pistachios
Corn	Eel	Pumpkin seeds
Garbanzo beans	Flatfish	Sesame seeds
Green beans	Haddock	Sunflower seeds
Kidney beans	Halibut	Walnuts
Leeks	Herring	
Lentils	Lamb	Fruits
Lima beans	Lobster	Apricots
Navy beans	Mackerel	Avocado
Okra	Oysters	Banana
Parsnips	Perch	Cantaloupe
Peas	Pike	Currants
Pinto beans	Salmon	Figs
Potatoes	Scallops	Grapefruit juice
Pumpkin	Shrimp	Orange juice
Soybean sprouts	Snapper	Papaya
Spinach	Trout	Pineapple juice
Squash	Turkey	Prunes
Yams		Raisins

Grains
Brown rice
Millet
Wild rice

7

Stress Reduction for Relief of Endometriosis

Many of the endometriosis patients I see in my medical practice complain of major stress along with their physical symptoms. My personal impression as a physician is that stress is a significant component of many recurrent and chronic health problems, including endometriosis. To discount the effects of lifestyle stress on illness is a grave mistake. If the physician ignores stress as a contributing factor, the patient never receives the tools or insight necessary to modify her habits and behavior to better support good health and well-being.

Research studies have confirmed the negative effects of stress on many different diseases. On the physiological level, stress increases the cortisone output from the adrenal glands, impairs immune function, elevates blood pressure and heart rate, and affects hormonal balance. In women with endometriosis, stress may negatively affect hormonal balance and muscle tone, upsetting the estrogen and progesterone balance and triggering excessive output of adrenal stress hormones. This can impair the body's ability to limit the scarring and inflammation caused by the endometrial implants.

Stress in endometriosis patients can arise over such issues as job security and performance, money worries, relationship problems with family and friends, overwork, and a host of other common problems. In addition, women with endometriosis have specific stress due to the diseases themselves, including concerns about their health and about the painful symptoms that are disrupting their lives and well-being. The infertility that can result from endometriosis is a particularly upsetting problem for women who are trying to start a family. The pain during intercourse that is also common in women with endometriosis can disrupt a healthy sexual relationship, causing anguish and discord.

A variety of stress management techniques can help women suffering from endometriosis. Some women find counseling or psychotherapy to be effective, while others depend heavily on the support of family and friends. Many women find it helpful to rethink their way of handling stressful situations and to implement lifestyle changes. Practicing stress-reduction techniques like meditation and deep-breathing exercises on a regular basis also helps them handle stress more effectively, as does a program of physical exercise. Whatever methods you decide to practice, I urge you to look at your stress level carefully and make every effort to handle emotionally-charged issues as calmly as possible.

The stress management exercises described in this chapter are a very important part of the endometriosis self-help program I recommend to my patients. For many women, the intensity of menstrual pain and cramps varies from month to month, depending on many lifestyle factors. My patients frequently tell me their bleeding and cramps are worse when they are more upset. As you begin to anticipate the onset of your menstrual period, I recommend using stress-reduction techniques on a daily basis. They can really make a difference. If you break up the tasks of the day with a few minutes of stress-reducing exercises, you will feel much more relaxed. With the use of these stress-reduction techniques, you can accomplish tasks on time but in a much more relaxed, enjoyable, and health-enhancing manner.

Exercises for Relaxation

To help you cope with the emotional stresses that may become magnified if you are suffering from endometriosis related symptoms, I recommend a variety of relaxation methods. Focusing, meditation, muscle relaxation, affirmations, and visualizations can each help foster a sense of calm and well-being if practiced on a regular basis. This chapter includes exercises from all of these categories for you to try. Pick those you enjoy most and practice them on a regular basis. I have taught these exercises to women patients for many years and love to practice them myself. Sometimes I recommend that my patients learn these techniques on their own through books and tapes; other times I teach the exercises to patients at my office.

My patients have been very enthusiastic about the results they attain through stress-reduction exercises. They often tell me that they feel much calmer and happier. They also find their physical health improves. A calm mind seems to have beneficial effects on the body's physiology and chemistry, restoring the body to a normal condition.

To prepare yourself for the relaxation exercises in this chapter, I suggest taking the following steps:

First Step. Wear loose, comfortable clothes. Find a comfortable position. For many women, this means lying on their backs. You may also do the exercises sitting up. Try to make your spine as straight as possible. Uncross your arms and legs.

Second Step. Focus your attention on the exercises. Do not allow thoughts to distract you and interfere with your concentration. Close your eyes and take a few deep breaths, in and out. This will help remove your thoughts from the problems and tasks of the day and begin to quiet your mind.

Exercise 1: Focusing

If you have endometriosis-related menstrual cramps and pelvic pain, this focusing exercise takes your attention off your pelvic region and lower part of your body as you focus elsewhere, clearing your mind and breathing deeply. At the end of this exercise, you may find that your discomfort is less severe. This is also a helpful exercise for inducing a sense of peace and calm.

- Sit upright in a comfortable position.

- Hold your watch in the palm of your hand.

- Focus all of your attention on the movements of the second hand of the watch.

- Inhale and exhale as you do this. Continue to concentrate for 30 seconds. Don't let any other thoughts enter your mind. At the end of this time, notice your breathing. You will probably find that it has slowed down and is calmer. You may also feel a sense of peacefulness and a decrease in any anxiety that you had on beginning this exercise.

Exercise 2: Peaceful Meditation

Many women suffering from endometriosis complain of daily life stresses. Stress can lower the pain threshold, increasing muscle tension and discomfort. It can also worsen PMS-related irritability and mood swings, which often coexist with endometriosis. Simple meditation techniques are a way to combat this stress.

Meditation requires you to sit quietly and engage in a simple and repetitive activity. By emptying your mind, you give yourself a rest. The metabolism of your body slows down. Meditating gives your mind a break from tension and worry. It is particularly useful during menstruation, when every little stress is magnified. After meditating you may find your mood greatly improved and your ability to handle everyday stress enhanced.

- Lie or sit in a comfortable position.

- Close your eyes and breathe deeply. Let your breathing be slow and relaxed.

- Focus all of your attention on your breathing. Notice the movement of your chest and abdomen in and out.

- Block out all other thoughts, feelings, and sensations. If you feel your attention wandering, bring it back to your breathing.

- Say the word "rest" as you inhale. Say the word "relax" as you exhale. Draw out the pronunciation of each word so that it lasts for the entire breath: r-r-r-r-e-e-e-e-s-s-s-s-t-t-t-t, r-r-r-e-e-e-l-l-l-a-a-a-x-x-x. Repeating these two words will help you to concentrate.

- Repeat this exercise until you feel very relaxed.

Exercise 3: Healing Meditation

This meditation exercise promotes healing through a series of beautiful and peaceful images you can invoke to create a positive mental state during your premenstrual and menstrual time of the month. (You can use this exercise during your symptom-free time, too.)

The premise of a healing meditation is the fact that the mind and body are inextricably linked. When you visualize a beautiful scene in which your body is being healed, you stimulate positive chemical and hormonal changes that help to create this condition. This process can reduce pain, discomfort, and irritability. Likewise, if you visualize a negative scene, such as a fight with a spouse or a boss, the negative mental picture can trigger an output of chemicals in the body that can worsen the symptoms caused by endometriosis. The axiom "you are what you think" is literally true. I have seen the power of positive thinking for years in my medical practice. I always tell my patients that healing the body is much harder if the mind is full of upset, angry, or fearful images. Healing meditations, when practiced on a regular basis, can be a powerful therapeutic tool. If you enjoy this form of meditation, try designing your own with images that make you feel good.

- Lie on your back in a comfortable position. Inhale and exhale slowly and deeply.

- Visualize a beautiful green meadow full of lovely fragrant flowers. In the middle of this meadow is a golden temple. See the temple emanating peace and healing.

- Visualize yourself entering this temple. You are the only person inside. It is still and peaceful. As you stand inside this temple, you feel a healing energy fill every pore of your body with a warm golden light. This energy feels like a healing balm that relaxes you totally. All anxiety dissolves and fades from your mind. You feel totally at ease.

- Open your eyes and continue your deep, slow breathing for another minute.

Exercise 4: Discovering Muscle Tension

This and the following exercise help you get in touch with your areas of muscle tension, and then teach you how to release that tension. This is an important sequence for women with endometriosis who suffer from recurrent menstrual cramps, low back pain, or abdominal discomfort. Many of these symptoms are due in part to the chronically tight and tense muscles that can accompany endometriosis. Tense muscles tend to have decreased blood circulation and oxygenation, and may accumulate an excess of waste products like carbon dioxide and lactic acid.

Interestingly enough, some women with menstrual cramps and pelvic pain carry tension in these areas throughout the month, even when cramps are absent. They tend to tighten the pelvic and lower abdominal muscles in response to work, relationship, and sexual stresses. Usually, this tensing of the pelvic muscles is an unconscious response that develops over many years and sets up the emotional patterning that triggers cramps. For example, when a woman has uncomfortable feelings about sex or a particular sexual partner, she may tighten these muscles when engaging in or even thinking about sex. Tense muscles also affect a woman's moods, making her more "uptight" and irritable.

Muscular and emotional tensions usually coexist. Movement is one effective way of breaking up these habitual patterns of muscle holding and contracting. When muscles are loose and limber, a woman tends to feel more relaxed and in a better mood. Anxiety tends to fade away, replaced by a sense of expansiveness and calm.

- Lie in a comfortable position. Allow your arms to rest comfortably by your sides, palms down, on the surface next to you.

- Now, raise just the right hand and arm and hold it elevated for 15 seconds.

- Notice if your forearm feels tight and tense or if the muscles are soft and pliable.

- Now, let your hand and arm drop down and relax. The arm muscles will relax too.

- As you lie still, notice any other parts of your body that feel tense, any muscles that feel tight and sore. You may notice a constant dull aching in certain muscles. Tense muscles block blood flow and cut off the supply of nutrients to the tissues. In response to the poor oxygenation, the muscle produces lactic acid, which further increases muscular discomfort.

Exercise 5: Progressive Muscle Relaxation

- Lie in a comfortable position. Allow your arms to rest at your sides, palms down, on the surface next to you.

- Inhale and exhale slowly and deeply.

- Clench your hands into fists and hold them tightly for 15 seconds. As you do this, relax the rest of your body. Visualize the tense part contracting, becoming tighter and tighter.

- Then let your hands relax. On relaxing, see a golden light flowing into the entire body, making all your muscles soft and pliable.

- Now, tense and relax the following parts of your body in this order: face, shoulders, back, stomach, pelvis, legs, feet, and toes. Hold each part tensed for 15 seconds and then relax your body for 30 seconds before going on to the next part.

- Finish the exercise by shaking your hands and imagining the remaining tension flowing out of your fingertips.

Exercise 6: Affirmations

Affirmations are positive statements that describe how you want your body to be. They are very important because they align your mind with your body in a positive way. As the healing meditations (exercise 3) achieve this goal through the use of positive images, affirmations do it through the power of suggestion. Your state of health is determined in part by the interaction between your mind and body via the thousands of messages you send yourself each day with your thoughts.

You can aggravate your endometriosis menstrual bleeding and cramps as well as pelvic discomfort with negative thoughts; because when your body believes it is sick, it behaves accordingly. Thus, it is essential to cultivate a positive belief system and a positive body image as part of your healing program. It is not enough to follow an excellent diet and a vigorous exercise routine when you are in the process of healing menstrual cramps. You must also tell your body that it is a well, fully functional system. I have seen people stay ill and sabotage their healing program by sending themselves a barrage of negative messages.

Sit in a comfortable position. Repeat the following affirmations. Repeat three times those that are particularly important to you.

- My female system is strong and healthy.

- My hormonal levels are perfectly balanced and regulated.

- My body chemistry is healthy and balanced.

- I go through my monthly menstrual cycle with ease and comfort.

- My menstrual flow self-regulates. I have light to moderate bleeding.

- My body is relaxed and pain-free.

- My vaginal muscles are relaxed and comfortable.

- My cervix and uterus are relaxed and pain-free.

- My uterus is normal in size and shape.

- My menstrual flow leaves my body easily and effortlessly each month.

- My body feels wonderful as I start each monthly period.

- I barely know that my body is getting ready to menstruate.

- I feel wonderful each month before I menstruate.

- My uterus is relaxed and receptive; I welcome my monthly period.

- My low back muscles feel supple and pliable with each menstrual cycle.

- I am relaxed and at ease as my period approaches.

- I desire a well-balanced and healthful diet.

- I eat only the foods that are good for my female body

- It is a real pleasure to take good care of my body

- I do the level of exercise that keeps my body healthy and supple.

- I handle stress easily and in a relaxed manner.

- I love my body; I feel at ease in my body.

- My body is pain-free and relaxed.

Exercise 7: Visualizations

Visualization exercises help you lay down the mental blueprint for a healthier body. This powerful technique can stimulate positive chemical and hormonal changes in your body to help create the desired outcome. Through positive visualization, you are imaging your body the way you want it to function and be. The body can modify its chemical and hormonal output in response to this technique and move toward a state of improved health. As a result, you may find this technique useful for reducing the symptoms and severity of both endometriosis.

Patients with many types of illnesses have used visualization to great benefit. The technique was pioneered by Carl Simonton, M.D., a cancer radiation therapist who used visualization with his patients. Aware that his patients tended to see their cancer as a "big destructive monster," he had them instead visualize their immune systems as big white knights or white sharks attacking the small and insignificant cancer cells and destroying them (instead of the other way around). In many cases, he saw his patients' health improve.

This visualization exercise for endometriosis uses an "erasure" image that helps you see your endometrial implants melt away and disappear. Simply skip the part of the exercise that does not pertain to your symptoms.

- Sit in a comfortable position.

- Close your eyes. Begin to breathe deeply. Inhale and let the air out slowly. Feel your body begin to relax.

- Imagine that you can look, as if through a magic mirror, deep inside your own body.

- Focus on any areas of your reproductive tract that you sense contain endometrial implants. See any lesions, cysts, or scarring that the endometriosis has caused. You may visualize the actual implants, or you may simply see the endometriosis as discolored areas within your body (colors such as gray or brown are common).

- Next, imagine a large eraser, like the kind used to erase chalk marks, coming into your pelvic area. See this eraser rubbing the areas of endometriosis. See these implants begin to loosen, shrink, and finally disappear.

- Now, look at your female organs. See your uterus and ovaries. They are an attractive pink color. Your uterus is relaxed and supple. Your uterus is becoming its normal size and shape. Your uterus has good blood circulation. Look at your ovaries. They are extremely healthy and put out just the right levels of hormones. They are shiny and pink and look like two almonds. The fallopian tubes that pick up the eggs and bring them to the uterus are totally open and healthy.

- Look at your abdominal and low back muscles. They are soft and pliable with a healthy muscle tone. They are relaxed and free of tension during your menstrual period. Your abdomen is flat and your fluid balance is perfect in your pelvic area.

- Look at your entire body and enjoy the sense of peace and calm running through your body. You feel wonderful.

- Stop visualizing the scene, and focus on your deep breathing, inhaling and exhaling slowly

- You open your eyes and feel very good. Visualizing this scene should take a minute or two. Linger on any images that particularly please you.

More Stress-Reduction Techniques

The rest of this chapter explains other techniques that I have found useful for relaxing tight and tense muscles. You can also use these methods to induce deep emotional relaxation. Try them for a delightful experience.

Hydrotherapy

For centuries, people have used warm water to relax their muscles and calm their mood. You can create your own "spa" at home by adding relaxing ingredients to the bath water. I have found two recipes extremely useful in relieving muscle pain and tension related to endometriosis.

Recipe 1: Alkaline Bath. Run a tub of warm water. Heat will increase your menstrual flow, so keep the water a little cooler if that is a problem. Add one cup of sea salt and one cup of bicarbonate of soda to the tub. As this is a highly alkaline mixture, I recommend using it only once or twice a month. I've found it very helpful in reducing cramps and calming anxiety and irritability. Soak for 20 minutes. You will probably feel relaxed and sleepy after this bath. Try it at night before going to sleep. You will probably wake up feeling refreshed and energized the following day. Heat of any kind helps to release muscle tension. You may also want to try a hot water bottle or a heating pad to relieve cramps.

Recipe 2: Hydrogen Peroxide Bath. This is one of my personal favorites. Hydrogen peroxide is a combination of water and oxygen, by adding it to your bath, you "hyper-oxygenate" the water. This helps to induce muscle relaxation. Hydrogen peroxide is inexpensive and can be purchased from your local drug store or supermarket. I usually add three pint bottles of the 3-percent solution to a full tub of warm water and soak for up to 30 minutes. If you use the stronger food- or technical-grade hydrogen peroxide (35 percent strength), add only 6 ounces. With the more concentrated peroxide, be sure to avoid direct contact with your hands or eyes and keep it stored in a cool place, as it is a very powerful oxidizer.

Sound

Music can have a tremendously relaxing effect on our minds and bodies. For women with endometriosis-related cramps and pain, I recommend slow, quiet music—classical music is particularly good. This type of music can have a pronounced beneficial effect on your physiological functions. It can slow your pulse and heart rate, lower your blood pressure, and decrease your levels of stress hormones. It can also help reduce anxiety and induce sleep for women with cramps. Equally beneficial are nature sounds, such as ocean waves and rainfall; these sounds can also induce a sense of peace and relaxation. I have patients who keep tapes of nature sounds in their car and at home for use when they feel stressed. Play relaxing music often as your menstrual cycle approaches and you are aware of increased levels of emotional and physical tension.

Biofeedback Therapy

Biofeedback therapy is an effective way to relieve pain of all kinds caused by muscular tension, as well as poor circulation caused by narrowing of the blood-vessel diameter. Constriction of the skeletal muscles and the smooth muscle of the blood-vessel wall usually occurs on an unconscious basis, so a person is not even aware that it's happening. A variety of factors, including emotional stress and nutritional or chemical imbalances, can trigger this involuntary muscle tension. This constriction can worsen problems such as endometriosis, fibroid tumors, migraine headaches, and high blood pressure.

Using biofeedback therapy, people learn to recognize when they are tensing their muscles. Once this response is understood, endometriosis sufferers can learn to relax their muscles to help relieve the pain. Since muscle relaxation both decreases muscular discomfort and improves blood flow, either factor can be monitored. For relief of cramps, women can learn how to implement biofeedback therapy through a series of training sessions, requiring about 10 to 15 thirty-minute office visits with a trained professional. During these sessions, a thermometer is inserted into the vagina like a tampon. The thermometer is connected to a digital readout machine that monitors the woman's internal temperature. The professional teaches her how to consciously change her vaginal temperature. Even a slight rise in the temperature indicates better blood flow and muscle relaxation in the pelvic area, with a concomitant relief of menstrual pain.

After the training sessions, most women are able to raise their temperature at will and thereby control their own cramps. I went through biofeedback training many years ago and found that it had a significant effect on my level of muscle tension. Many hospitals and university centers have biofeedback units, as do stress management clinics, so it is relatively easy to find a treatment facility that offers this type of therapy.

Putting Your Stress-Reduction Program Together

This chapter has introduced many different ways to reset your mind and body to help make menstruation a calm and relaxed time of the month and ease the symptoms of endometriosis. Try each exercise at least once. Experiment with them until you find the combination that works for you. Doing all seven exercises will take no longer than 20 to 30 minutes, depending on how much time you wish to spend with each one. Ideally, you should do the exercises at least a few minutes each day. Over time, they will help you gain insight into your negative beliefs and change them into positive new ones. Your ability to cope with stress should improve tremendously.

8

Breathing Exercises

Breathing exercises are a simple yet powerful way to reduce endometriosis-related pain and cramps. Through therapeutic breathing, you can relax and loosen your muscles, decrease sensations of pain, lower your anxiety level, and generate a feeling of internal peace and calm. This process grants you a degree of voluntary control over your discomfort. Many of my patients find the combination of breathing exercises and stress-reduction techniques to be very empowering.

When you are breathing slowly and deeply, you take large amounts of oxygen into your circulatory system, where it binds to the red blood cells as it travels through the arteries and veins. Oxygen enables the cells to produce and utilize energy, and to remove waste products through the production of carbon dioxide. These waste products are cleared through exhalation by the lungs. Thus, the whole body needs optimal levels of oxygen for its normal cycle of building, repair, and elimination. Although there are no specific studies on the use of breathing exercises in patients with endometriosis, I believe that the stress-reducing benefits may help your body limit and repair the damage caused by endometriosis.

When you are in physical and emotional distress, oxygen levels decrease. Breathing tends to become jagged, erratic, and shallow.

You may find yourself breathing too fast or with severe pain. You may stop breathing altogether and hold your breath for prolonged periods of time without even realizing it. None of these breathing patterns is healthful. Anxious breathing is often linked to other unhealthy physiological reactions that reflect your body's state of stress. When you have cramps and pain, besides lowering the oxygen level in your body, you tend to tighten your muscles, constrict blood flow, elevate your pulse rate and heartbeat, and stimulate the output of stressful chemicals from your glands in response to the pelvic discomfort. Waste products like carbon dioxide and lactic acid also accumulate in your muscles and other tissues.

Therapeutic breathing exercises provide a way to break up this pattern and help the body return to equilibrium. It is important to do the breathing exercises in a slow and regular manner. First, find a comfortable position. Some exercises you should do lying on your back; for other exercises, you'll sit up, uncross your arms and legs, and keep your back straight.

Exercise 1: Deep Abdominal Breathing

Deep, slow abdominal breathing is an important technique for the relief of endometriosis-related cramps and pain. It brings adequate oxygen, the fuel for metabolic activity, to all the tissues of your body. Rapid, shallow breathing decreases your oxygen supply and keeps you devitalized. Deep breathing helps relax the entire body and strengthens the muscles in the chest and abdomen. It also helps calm many other physiological processes, such as the rapid pulse rate and heartbeat that often accompany menstrual cramps.

- Lie flat on your back with your knees pulled up. Keep your feet slightly apart. Try to breathe in and out through your nose.

- Inhale deeply. As you breathe in, allow your stomach to relax so that the air flows into your abdomen. Your stomach should balloon out as you breathe in. Visualize your lungs filling up with air so that your chest swells out.

- Imagine that the air you breathe is filling your body with energy.

- Exhale deeply. As you breathe out, let your stomach and chest collapse. Imagine the air being pushed out, first from your abdomen and then from your lungs.

Exercise 2: Peaceful, Slow Breathing

Breathing slowly and peacefully can actually decrease anxiety and help promote a sense of inner calm and quiet. Such breathing helps our mind to slow down and our emotions become happier and more harmonious. Life feels good. When we are calm, we make better decisions and relate to those around us in a healthier way.

Breathing slowly can also calm our physical responses by helping to balance autonomic nervous system function. The autonomic nervous system regulates functions that we're usually not aware of, such as circulation of the blood, muscle tension, pulse rate, breathing, and glandular function. The autonomic nervous system is divided into two parts that oppose and complement each other, the sympathetic and parasympathetic systems.

The sympathetic nervous system is linked to tension and the "fight-or-flight" response of fear and panic, while the parasympathetic nervous system regulates body responses that are relaxed and calm. When women have menstrual cramps and low back pain, the sympathetic nervous system is in overdrive. The pain sensation causes muscles to tense.

Furthermore, the pulse rate tends to accelerate and the blood vessels to constrict. Slow, peaceful breathing is a way to calm down these stress responses and bring the body back to a state of balance. By slowing down our breathing, we slow down our other physiologic responses. Our muscles relax and our blood vessels dilate; we have restored a state of equilibrium.

- Lie flat on your back with your knees pulled up. Keep your feet slightly apart. Try to breathe in and out through your nose.

- Inhale deeply. As you breathe in, allow your stomach to relax so that the air flows into your abdomen. Let your stomach balloon out as you breathe in. Visualize the lowest parts of your lungs filling up with air.

- Imagine that the air you are breathing in is filled with peace and calm. A sensation of peace and calm is filling every cell of your body. Your whole body feels warm and relaxed as you breathe in this air. Now, exhale deeply. As you breathe out, imagine the air being pushed out from the bottom of your lungs to the top.

- Repeat this sequence until your entire body feels relaxed and your breathing is slow and regular.

Exercise 3: Grounding

Women suffering from pain and discomfort due to endometriosis can lose a sense of being grounded, or rooted to the earth. Some women report a sensation of numbness in their legs and feet or feel as if they have no legs at all. This is due in part to the fact that endometriosis-related pelvic cramps and low back pain cause leg muscles to tighten and blood circulation and oxygenation to the lower extremities to decrease.

If you are feeling ungrounded focusing and concentrating can be difficult. You may have difficulty sitting at a desk and working through your projects for the day in a coherent manner. This exercise will help you to ground and focus both physically and mentally. You should feel much more stable and focused by the end of this exercise.

Sit upright in a chair. Be sure you are in a comfortable position. Keep your feet slightly apart. Breathe in and out through your nose.

- Inhale deeply. As you breathe in, allow your stomach to relax so that the air flows into your abdomen. Let your stomach balloon out as you breathe in. Visualize the lowest parts of your lungs filling up with air. Hold your inhalation.

- Visualize a golden cord with a golden ball at the end of it running from the base of your spine. Let this golden cord gently and slowly move downwards through the earth, grounding you. You can let it move down as far as you would like, even all the way to the center of the earth.

- Follow the cord and its golden ball in your mind all the way down and see it fasten securely to the earth's center. You can run two golden cords from the bottoms of your feet down to the center of the earth, also, if you would like.

- As you exhale, become aware of your hips, thighs, calves, ankles, and feet. Feel their strength and solidity.

- Repeat this exercise several times until you feel fully present and grounded.

Exercise 4: Muscle-Tension Release Breathing

This exercise will help you get in touch with and release general muscle tension and tightness. Often when the uterus, abdominal muscles, and low back are tight, you unconsciously tense up muscles throughout your entire body, making the neck, shoulders, and other vulnerable areas tense, too. You can have tense muscles in other parts of the body without being aware of it. This exercise will help you focus on any tension that you are carrying in your upper body. It will also help you take your focus off your cramps. As you relax and release the muscles in your neck and shoulders, you will also release muscle tension in your entire body. This is a good exercise to do while walking, engaging in sports, or taking care of desk work, to get in touch with any muscle tension you may be carrying.

- Sit upright in a chair. (If you perform this exercise while walking or involved in another activity, just be in a position that is as comfortable as possible.) Be sure you are in a comfortable position. Keep your feet slightly apart. Try to breathe in and out through your nose.

- Inhale and exhale deeply. As you breathe, let your head move from side to side. Keep your shoulders down and try to touch your ear to your shoulder. As you do this movement, imagine that your neck is made out of putty, allowing your head to move in a supple, relaxed movement from left to right.

- Now inhale and pull your shoulders up toward your ears. Hold your breath and keep your shoulders in a hunched position. Exhale and let your shoulders drop back into a relaxed, comfortable position. Repeat this several times.

- Inhale and exhale deeply as you roll your shoulders forward. Make a large, slow, circular motion with your shoulders. Then, roll your shoulders back slowly. Repeat this several times.

- Inhale and exhale deeply, keeping the rest of your body still and relaxed. Repeat this several times.

Exercise 5: Emotional Cleansing Breath

During my years of medical practice, I have seen menstrual cramps, inflammatory pain, and even menstrual bleeding problems intensify when women are under emotional stress. The more day-to-day stress you have over family, work, and other personal issues, the more this can aggravate your endometriosis. In fact, many of my patients have told me they believe that their unhealed personal relationships, as well as sexual problems, are significant emotional triggers for their cramps and pain.

This particular exercise uses breathing to help you release any negative feelings, chronic anger, or upset that you may be harboring. The more time you spend cleansing old negative emotional patterns, the less impact these feelings can have on your sensitive female reproductive tract with the onset of each menstruation.

- Lie flat on your back with your knees pulled up. Keep your feet slightly apart. Try to breathe in and out through your nose.

- Inhale deeply and see yourself enveloped in a soft white light. Breathe this light into every cell of your body. This is a cleansing light and can help wash away fear, anger, anxiety, and other negative feelings.

- As you exhale deeply, feel the light washing these emotions away.

- Repeat this exercise until you feel emotionally peaceful and clear.

Exercise 6: Color Breathing with Red

Color breathing (Exercises 6 and 7) has been used in more than one ancient tradition to heal the body and strengthen the body's energy field. Intuitives in our culture can see this energy field as light or colors emanating from the body. When a person is calm, relaxed, and healthy, the energy field looks radiant and full of colors. The colors are bright and harmonious, and each one corresponds to specific parts of the body.

When we are feeling pain or tension, as often happens with the chronic symptoms of endometriosis, we literally lose light and color. Our energy field looks more discordant and jagged, and the colors become duller, or muddied. Color breathing is a technique that can help strengthen and heal the energy field as well as the body itself. As you breathe in the healing colors, the parts of your body that are in pain and discomfort often begin to relax and feel healthier again. Tension and cramping is replaced by a sensation of lightness and peace.

- Sit or lie in a comfortable position. Take a deep breath and visualize that the earth below you is a deep scarlet red. Imagine that you are opening up energy centers on the bottoms of your feet.

- As you inhale, visualize the deep scarlet red color filling up your feet. Draw this color up your legs and into your pelvic area. See it first filling up your legs, then your lower back, and finally your pelvis. Your uterus is filling with a beautiful deep scarlet red color.

- As you exhale, see this color dissolving and washing away any areas of endometriosis in your body. See this color flow out of your uterus and lower back and fill the air around you. Exhale the deep scarlet red slowly out of your lungs. Repeat this process 5 times.

Exercise 7: Color Breathing with Golden Light

- Sit or lie in a comfortable position.

- Imagine a cloud of beautiful golden energy surrounding you. As you take a deep breath, inhale the golden energy and visualize it flowing through your body and into your uterus, pelvic area, and lower back. This is a healing energy—it warms and relaxes your uterus, lower abdominal muscles, and lower back.

- Hold the inhalation as long as it is comfortable. Let this golden cloud pick up all your pain and tension.

- Then, exhale this energy out through your lungs and let it be carried away from you.

- Repeat this process as many times as needed until the pain is replaced by a feeling of peace and calm.

9

Physical Exercises

Exercise is an important part of an endometriosis-relief program because of its role in pain relief and the prevention of the menstrual pain and cramps that accompany these conditions. To better understand how exercise can provide relief, let us look first at the physiological effects that endometriosis produces in your body. Many women with both conditions complain of pain and discomfort. This includes pain at mid-cycle, in the two weeks prior to the onset of menstruation, with sexual intercourse, and even with bowel movements and urination if the endometrial implants have invaded the neighboring organs. Endometriosis causes internal bleeding in the pelvis which worsens inflammation. Endometrial implants can impinge on nerves and neighboring organ systems and can cause inflammation and scarring in the pelvic tissues.

In response to the discomfort caused by these two conditions, women often involuntarily contract the muscles of the pelvis, low back, and uterus. This is a natural response to pain. Tight and tense uterine and back muscles have decreased blood flow and oxygenation. Waste products such as excessive carbon dioxide can accumulate in this physical environment and further worsen symptoms. In addition, the pain of menstrual cramps causes breathing to become rapid and shallow. Less oxygen is taken in through respiration, which further decreases the oxygen available to the pelvic region. Metabolism of the muscles becomes less efficient, and fluid retention can become a problem in the pelvic area as well as the ankles and feet. Many women complain of drawing pains in their thighs and aching sensations in their legs.

Aerobic exercise helps to relieve these symptoms. Playing tennis, walking, swimming, and dancing require deep breathing and active movement. With better respiration, oxygenation and blood flow to the pelvic area improve. The vigorous pumping action of the muscles that occurs with these activities helps reduce the congestive symptoms of menstrual cramps by moving blood and other fluids from the pelvic region. Exercise of this type should not, however, be done too vigorously. "Going for the burn" is not a good idea for women with endometriosis. Muscle fatigue from over exercise causes muscles to become oxygen-deficient and use up their reserve energy stores. This can intensify the pain symptoms of endometriosis.

Exercise also produces significant psychological benefits to sufferers of endometriosis. Improved oxygenation and blood flow benefit the brain as well as the pelvic muscles. For optimal functioning, the brain demands a healthy share of the body's available nutrients. When the brain and nervous systems are functioning well, exercise triggers an increased output of endorphins. These chemicals made by the brain have a natural opiate effect. Endorphins are thought to produce the "runner's high" that marathoners experience. Many women patients tell me that moderate and relaxed exercise is their most effective form of stress management, and that exercise produces a sense of peace and tranquility unmatched by anything else they do.

Another way aerobic exercise might help to reduce anxiety and calm the mood is by helping balance the autonomic nervous system. The autonomic nervous system regulates the "fight-or-flight" response that many women experience around the time of their menstrual period. When this system is in overdrive, small life worries can become magnified out of proportion because the body reacts to these small stresses as if they were life-threatening issues. Regular exercise helps lessen the intensity of this response. This can be a real benefit for endometriosis sufferers, many of whom lead complex and demanding lives.

I also recommend that women with endometriosis related menstrual cramps and low back pain consider doing flexibility and stretching exercises as part of their physical activity program. These exercises help prevent cramps and low back pain by strengthening the back and abdominal muscles. By balancing muscle tension through controlled, slow movement, stretching can also help to improve posture. When done properly, stretching exercises bring an awareness of how the parts of the body are aligned spatially with respect to each other.

In summary, exercise brings many healthful benefits to women who suffer from the symptoms of endometriosis. I recommend that women with these problems follow a regular program of physical activity for cramps throughout the entire month. Though exercise does not cure endometriosis, it can help alleviate both the physical and emotional symptoms that accompany these conditions. The remainder of this chapter describes a sequence of stretches and exercises useful in the relief of menstrual distress.

General Fitness and Flexibility Exercises

As part of your self-help program, the following set of exercises are good for mobility, flexibility, and relaxation. You can use them with great benefit during the premenstrual and menstrual time of the month to help loosen the joints in your lower body and decrease muscle stiffness and tension. You can also do these exercises throughout the month. Practiced on a regular basis, they will improve your vigor and energy level. The same exercises can help warm up tense and tight muscles before you engage in sports or athletic events.

I do many of these exercises myself and have found them to be very helpful during times of physical and emotional stress and tension. They have helped me tremendously to stay loose and flexible.

The following guidelines will help you perform the exercises safely and efficiently, without undue stress.

During the first week or two of your program, try all these exercises. Then put together your own routine based on the exercises that provide the most benefit. You may find that you want to use all of them on a regular basis or perhaps only a few of them. Warm-ups should always precede any sports or athletic event.

- Perform the exercises in a relaxed and unhurried manner. Be sure to set aside adequate time—about 30 minutes—so you do not feel rushed. Your work area should be quiet, peaceful, and uncluttered.

- Wear loose, comfortable clothing. It is better to exercise without socks to give your feet complete freedom of movement and to prevent slipping.

- Evacuate your bowels or bladder before you begin the exercises. Wait at least two hours after eating to exercise.

- Choose a flat area and work on a mat or a blanket. This will make you more comfortable while you do the exercises.

- When beginning an exercise, pay close attention to the initial instructions. Look at the placement of the body as shown in the photographs. This is very important, for you are much more likely to have relief of your symptoms if you do the exercise properly.

- Try to visualize the exercise in your mind, then follow with proper placement of the body.

- Move slowly through the exercise. This helps promote flexibility of the muscles and prevent injury.

- Always rest for a few minutes after doing the exercises.

- Try to practice these movements on a regular basis. A short session every day is best. If that is not possible, then try to practice them every other day.

Exercise 1: Deep Breathing

Deep, slow abdominal breathing is essential for women with endometriosis. It expands your lungs and allows you to bring adequate oxygen, the fuel for metabolic activity, to all the tissues of your body. Deep breathing will relax tight and contracted pelvic, abdominal, and low back muscles, thereby helping to relieve menstrual pain and distress. It also helps to relax the entire body and strengthens the muscles in the chest and abdomen. Deep breathing helps to stabilize mood and reduce both depression and anxiety, so it is very important for emotional well-being. In contrast, rapid, shallow breathing decreases your oxygen supply, which builds up lactic acid in the pelvic muscles, keeping them tense and tight.

Lie flat on your back with your knees pulled up. Keep your feet slightly apart. Try to breathe in and out through your nose.

Inhale deeply. As you breathe in, allow your stomach to relax so that the air flows into your abdomen. Your stomach should balloon out as you breathe in. Visualize your lungs filling up with air so that your chest swells out.

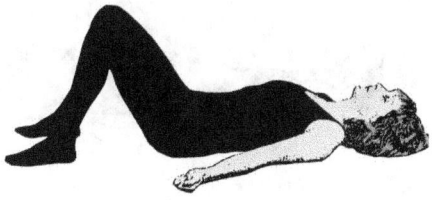

Imagine that the air you breathe is filling your body with energy

Exhale deeply. As you breathe out, let your stomach and chest collapse. Imagine the air being pushed out, first from your abdomen and then from your lungs.

Exercise 2: Total Body Muscle Relaxation

Women with endometriosis frequently have muscle groups that are tense and tight because of inadequate oxygenation and blood flow. Lactic acid tends to accumulate in these muscles, and muscle tension can become a chronic problem. This is particularly true during mid-cycle, at ovulation, and during the two weeks preceding menstruation. Shifts in the body's hormonal and mineral balance predispose women with these problems toward muscle tension.

Regular physical activity effectively breaks up this pattern of chronically tight muscles. During the second half of the menstrual cycle, it is very important to keep the muscles loose and flexible. Besides feeling more relaxed, supple muscles have a beneficial effect on the mood and induce an overall sense of peace and calm. The following exercise helps you to get in touch with the parts of your body that feel tense and contracted. It will also aid you in releasing muscle tension.

Lie in a comfortable position. Allow your arms to rest limply, palms down, on the surface next to you. Breathe slowly and deeply as you do this exercise.

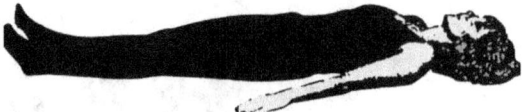

Raise your right hand off the floor and hold it there for 15 seconds. Notice any tension in your forearm or upper arm. Let your hand slowly relax and rest on the floor. The hand and arm muscles should relax. As you lie there, notice any other parts of your body where you are carrying tension.

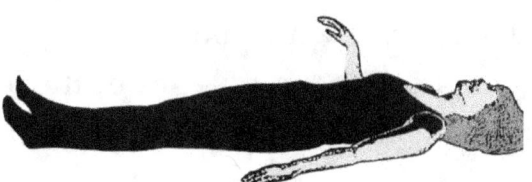

Clench your hands into fists and hold them tightly for 15 seconds. As you do this, relax the rest of your body. Then let your hands relax.

Now, tense and relax the following parts of your body in this order: face, shoulders, back, stomach, pelvis, legs, feet, and toes. Hold each part tensed for 15 seconds and then relax your body for 30 seconds before going on to the next part.

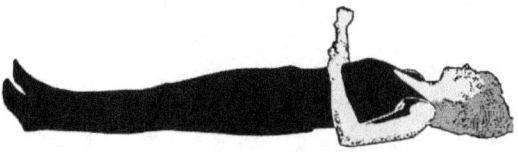

Visualize the tense part contracting, becoming tighter and tighter. On relaxing, see the energy flowing into the entire body like a gentle wave, making all the muscles soft and pliable.

Finish the exercise by shaking your hands. Imagine the remaining tension flowing out of your fingertips.

Exercise 3: Energizing Sequence

The pain and blood loss that accompany endometriosis can leave women feeling tired and depleted for several days to two weeks per month. This exercise sequence increases your energy, releases muscle tension, and improves circulation. The exercise stimulates movement and energy flow through all muscles of the body, starting from the legs and moving up to the top of the head. In traditional Indian healing models, these exercises are thought to stimulate the seven chakras or vital energy centers of the body. This sequence emphasizes the muscles of the lower extremities, low back, pelvis, and abdomen, since they are particularly affected by endometriosis.

Do the steps in this sequence slowly, so as not to stress the body. You will feel the benefits this exercise can have on your energy level if you don't rush through the steps or do them too hard. As your strength and flexibility improve, you may want to do the steps a little more vigorously.

Legs and Hips

Sit on the floor with your legs stretched straight in front of you. Place your hands on the floor behind you. Lift the buttocks off the floor and bounce gently on the base of your spine. Repeat 5 times.

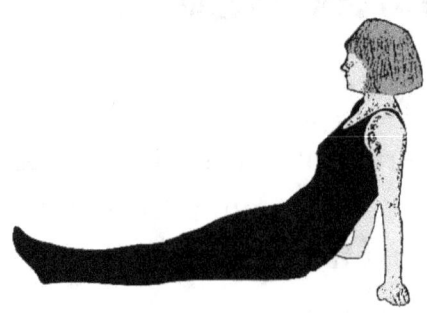

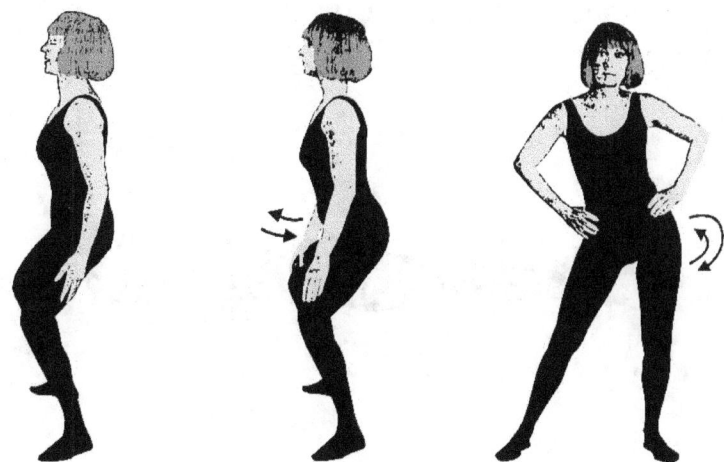

Stand with your legs spread apart about 2 feet. Point your feet out at a comfortable angle.

Rock your pelvis back and forth

Repeat 10 times. Then rotate your hips in a circular fashion, first moving clockwise and then counterclockwise.

Pelvis and Lower Abdomen

Lie on your stomach, placing your fists under your hips. Rest your forehead on the floor.

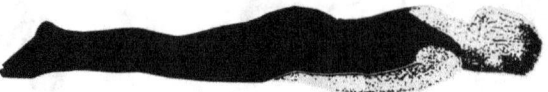

As you inhale, raise your right leg with an upward thrust, keeping your hips on your fists. Hold for 5 to 20 seconds if possible.

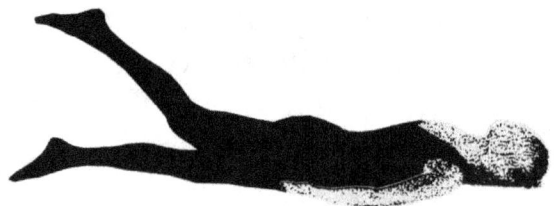

Lower the leg and slowly bring it back to the original position.

Repeat several times. Then do the exercise on the left side.

Abdomen and Chest

Sit on your heels with your hands placed on your knees. As you inhale, arch your back and stretch to expand your chest up and out.

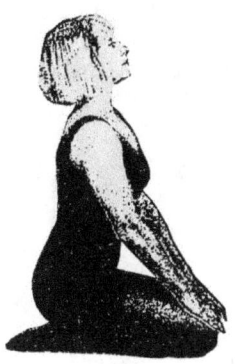

As you exhale, slump down to curve you back

Repeat several times

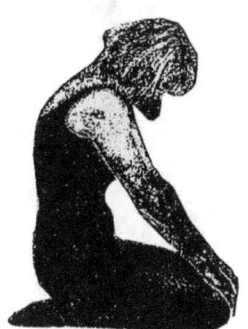

Exercise 4: Lower Back Arch

This exercise helps loosen the lower back muscles and improves flexibility of the spine. It can also combat tiredness in women who experience decreased energy during the onset of menstruation.

Stand with your legs spread 1 foot apart. Point your feet straight ahead.

Place your hands around your waist with your thumbs pressing into your lower back.

As you inhale, curve your back into an arch with your head held back.

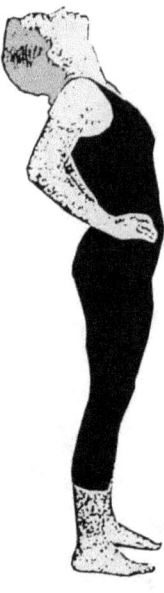

As you exhale, let the weight of your body bend you forward and curve in an arch, so that your head almost touches your knees. Hold this position for a few seconds.

Return to the original position as you inhale. Do this exercise slowly and repeat several times.

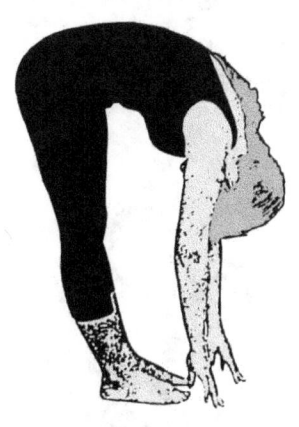

Exercise 5: Abdominal Muscle Release

This exercise helps to release lower and upper abdominal tension. Endometriosis implants may invade the bowel causing symptoms. This twist exercise helps reduce the tension in the abdominal muscles that can worsen these symptoms.

Sit on the floor with your legs out in front. Place your hands on your shoulders with your fingers in front and thumbs in back. Be sure to keep your spine straight and inhale deeply.

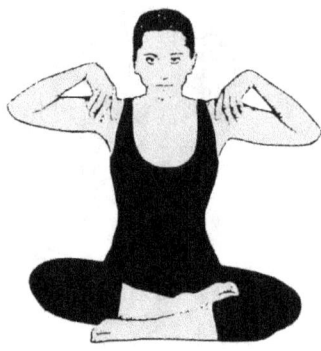

As you inhale, twist your head, chest, and abdomen to the left. As you exhale, twist your body to the right. Do this exercise 4 times. Then reverse directions and repeat the sequence.

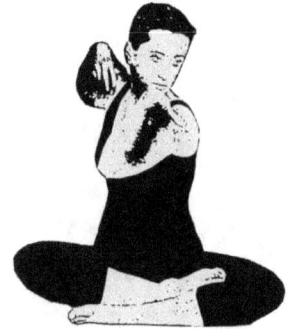 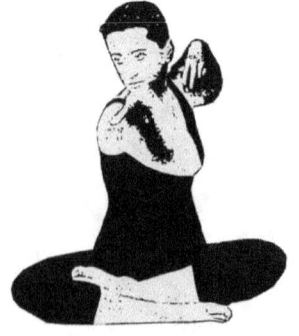

Exercise 6: Lower Back Release

This exercise promotes relaxation, specifically in the lower back, hips, and abdominal muscles. With the alternating tensing and releasing of the abdominal and hip muscles, along with controlled heavy breathing, the entire middle and lower body becomes looser and more supple. You may also notice a decrease in anxiety and emotional tension after this exercise.

Lie on your back with your legs together. Raise your feet 6 to 8 inches off the ground; then raise your head and shoulders 6 inches, also.

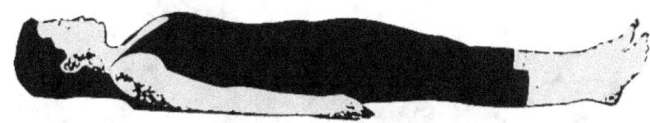

Point to your toes with your fingertips, keeping your arms straight and your eyes fixed on your toes. Then, breathe through your nose deeply to a count of 20.

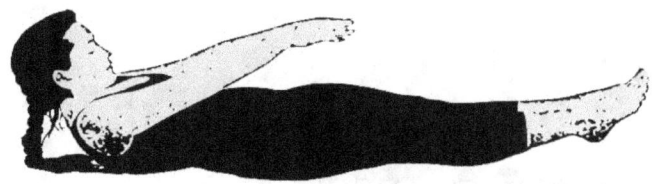

Lower your legs and head and relax. Rest for a count of 30. Repeat this exercise several times.

Exercise 7: Lower Back Twist

This exercise allows you to twist over to the side, which is actually a natural position for your body to assume when you are feeling pelvic discomfort. This gentle stretch helps to lengthen the muscles in the lower back as well as along the entire spine. It also helps to align the lumbar spine. Many women find that this exercise helps relieve pelvic tension and discomfort.

Lie on your back with your knees bent, feet placed flat on the floor.

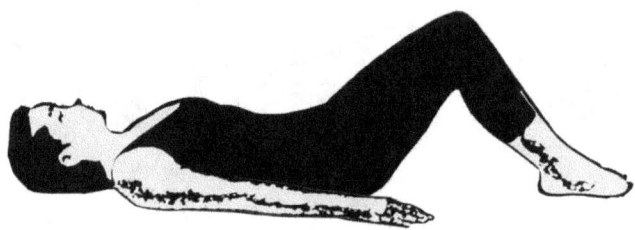

As you exhale, slowly let your knees and hips fall to the left as you turn your head to the right. Inhale and bring your knees back together to the center.

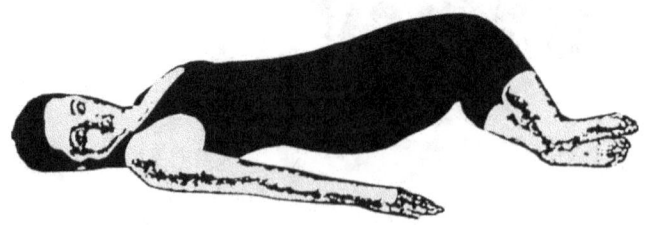

Then exhale again and reverse direction, letting your knees and hips fall to the right as you turn your head to the left.

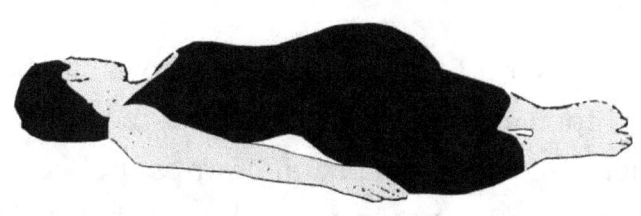

Repeat this exercise slowly several times, alternating sides.

10

Stretches for Relief of Endometriosis

The uncomfortable symptoms of endometriosis respond well to gentle stretches. Stretching exercises that emphasize pelvic movement and flexibility can help treat the menstrual cramps, pelvic congestion, and low back pain that commonly occur with this problem. Stretches may even help control heavy menstrual flow. The slow, controlled stretching movements that you do in these exercises help relax tense muscles and improve their suppleness and flexibility. They also bring better blood circulation and oxygenation to the tense areas of your lower body, thereby improving the metabolism of the pelvic and back muscles.

Stretches have an additional benefit in that it quiets your moods. The deep breathing and slow movements that characterize these exercises reduce anxiety and irritability and produce a sense of peace—a welcome change for women who have endometriosis and also have significant life stress. The stress reduction effects of stretches benefit all body systems, including the reproductive tract and the immune system.

In this chapter I present a series of specific stretches that gently stretch every muscle in your body, with specific emphasis on the pelvic and low back region. As well as relieving cramps and discomfort, these exercises energize and balance the female reproductive tract and can help correct underlying hormonal imbalance through improved oxygenation and better circulation to the pelvic area. This can have a beneficial effect on menstrual function. For women who are fatigued from the recurrent menstrual bleeding, pain, and discomfort these conditions cause, stretches can increase vigor and stamina. I do stretches frequently as part of my personal exercise routine.

When doing stretching exercises, it is important that you focus and concentrate on the positions. First, let your mind visualize how the pose is to look, and then follow with the correct body placement for the pose. Pay close attention to the initial instructions. Look at the placement of the body as shown in the photographs. This is very important, for if the pose is practiced properly, you are much more likely to have relief of your symptoms.

Be sure to move slowly through each pose. By taking it slowly, you have greater control over your body movements. You minimize the possibility of injury and maximize the benefit to the particular part of the body affected by the stretch. If you practice these stretches regularly in a slow, unhurried fashion, you will gradually loosen your muscles, ligaments, and joints. You may be surprised at how supple you can become over time.

If you experience any pain or discomfort, you have probably overreached your current ability and should immediately reduce the amount of stretching until you can proceed without discomfort. Be careful, as muscular injuries can take quite a while to heal. If you do strain a muscle, I have found that immediately applying ice to the injured area for 10 minutes is quite helpful. Continue to use the ice pack two to three times a day for several days. If the pain persists, see your doctor.

Follow the breathing instructions provided in the exercises. Most important, do not hold your breath. Allow your breath to flow in and out easily and effortlessly.

Stretch 1

This exercise helps stretch and release the low back and pelvic area. Besides relaxing this area and relieving pain, it also helps relieve hemorrhoids and constipation.

Sit on the floor with your legs placed straight out in front of you. Bend your right knee and place your right heel in your crotch area. Your left leg remains in a straight position.

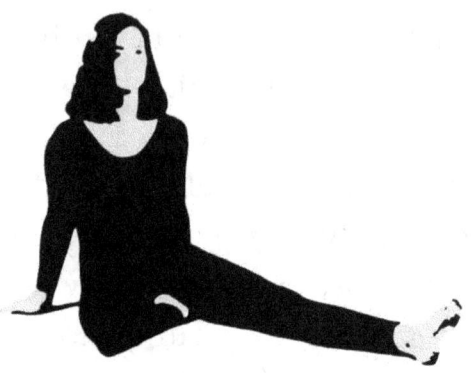

As you inhale, take hold of your left ankle, straightening your spine. Hold this position for 30 seconds.

As you exhale, bring your forehead toward your left knee. Hold this position for 30 seconds.

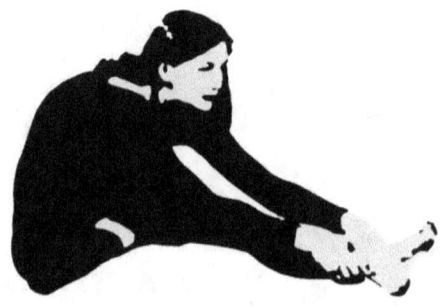

Stretch 2

This is an excellent exercise for stretching the abdominal muscles that are often tightened with menstrual cramps and pain caused by endometriosis. It is also helpful in reducing the pelvic congestion that occurs when PMS coexists with these conditions.

Lie on your back with your knees bent. Spread your feet apart, flat on the floor.

Place your hands around your ankles, holding them firmly.

As you inhale, arch your pelvis up and hold for a few seconds. As you exhale, relax and lower your pelvis.

Repeat this exercise several times.

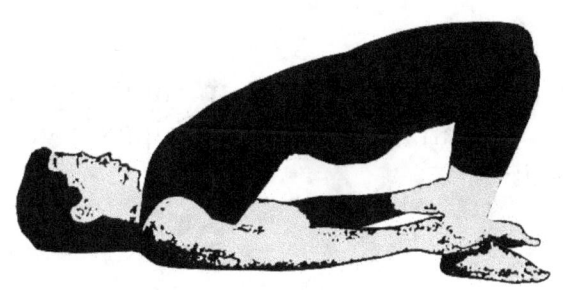

Stretch 3

This exercise strengthens the lower back, abdomen, buttocks, and legs, and relieves low back pain and menstrual cramps. It also energizes the entire female reproductive tract. Regular practice of this exercise helps improve posture and elimination and will tighten and firm the thighs and hips.

Lie face down on the floor. Make fists with both your hands and place them under your hips. This prevents compression of the lumbar spine while doing the exercise.

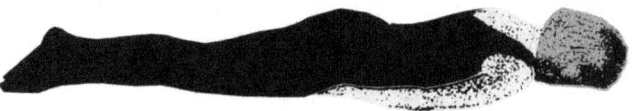

Straighten your body and raise your right leg with a slow upward thrust as high as you can, keeping your hips on your fists. Hold for 5 to 20 seconds if possible.

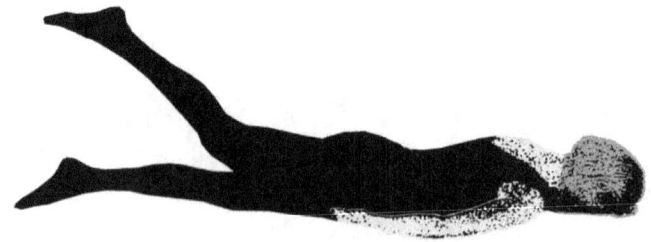

Lower the leg and slowly return to your original position. Repeat with the left leg, then with both legs together. Remember to keep your hips resting on your fists. Repeat 10 times.

Stretch 4

This exercise stretches the entire spine and helps relieve low back pain and menstrual cramps due to endometriosis. It stretches the abdominal muscles and strengthens the back, hips, and thighs. It also stimulates the digestive organs and endocrine glands. Regular practice of this posture can relieve depression and fatigue by improving your energy and elevating your mood.

Lie face down on the floor, arms at your sides. Slowly bend your legs at the knees and bring your feet up toward your buttocks.

Reach back with your arms and carefully take hold of first one foot and then the other. Flex your feet to make grasping them easier.

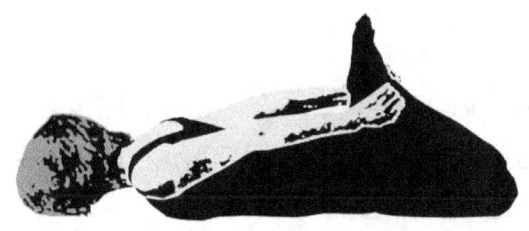

Inhale and raise your trunk from the floor as far as possible. Lift your head and elevate your knees off the floor.

Squeeze the buttocks. Imagine your body looking like a gently curved bow. Hold for 10 to 15 seconds.

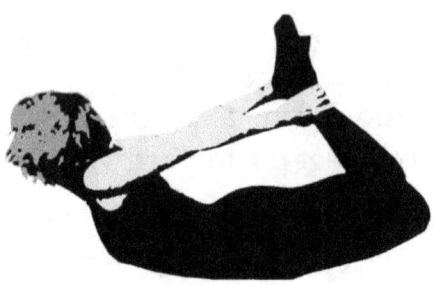

Slowly release the posture. Allow your chin to touch the floor and finally release your feet and return them slowly to the floor. Return to your original position. Repeat 5 times

Stretch 5

This exercise gently stretches the lower back. It is excellent for calming anxiety and irritability. Many of my patients with menstrual cramps practice this exercise often.

Sit on your heels. Bring your forehead to the floor, stretching the spine as far over your head as possible.

Close your eyes. Hold for as long as comfortable.

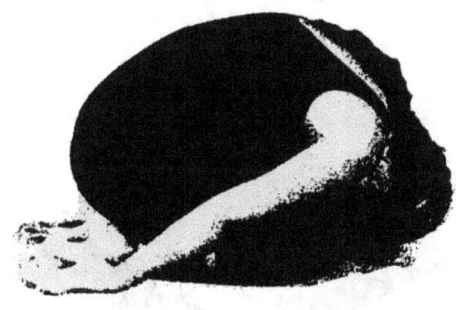

Stretch 6

This is another excellent exercise for menstrual related pain and cramps. It is also useful for reducing symptoms in women with coexisting PMS and helps to relieve the congestive symptoms that occur with menstrual cramps. This stretch opens the entire pelvic region and energizes the female reproductive tract; it also relieves bloating and fluid retention in legs and feet.

Lie on your back with your legs against the wall and extended out in a V or an arc, and your arms extended to the sides.

Hips should be as close to the wall as possible, buttocks on the floor. Spread legs apart as far as you can while still remaining comfortable.

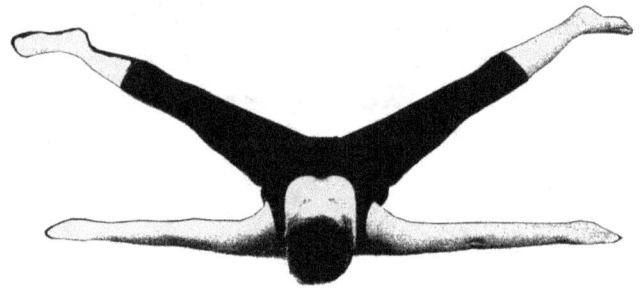

Breathing easily, hold for 1 minute, allowing the inner thighs to relax.

11

Acupressure Massage

Acupressure massage can help relieve the symptoms of bleeding, pain, and discomfort associated with endometriosis. It is based on an ancient Chinese healing method that applies finger pressure to specific points on the skin surface to prevent and treat illness. Acupressure has had a long and distinguished history as an effective healing tool for many centuries and is often used along with herbs to promote the healing of disease.

Though Traditional Chinese Medicine does not recognize the diagnoses of endometriosis, the symptoms of these conditions can nonetheless be alleviated by relieving the imbalances that they cause in the body, specifically in the flow of life energy, or chi. Chi is different from, yet similar to, electro-magnetic energy. According to this view, health is a state in which the chi is equally distributed throughout the body and is present in sufficient amounts. This occurs when there is a proper balance of yin (female) and yang (male) forces in the body. Chi, or life energy, is thought to energize all the cells and tissues of the body.

Traditional Chinese Medicine believes that chi runs through the body in channels called meridians. When working in a healthy manner, these channels distribute the energy evenly throughout the body, sometimes on the surface of the skin and at times deep inside the body, in the organs. When the energy flow in a meridian is blocked or stopped, disease occurs. As a result, the internal organs that correspond to the meridians can show symptoms of disease. Stimulating the points on the skin surface can correct the meridian flow. Hand massage can treat these points easily. Pressing specific acupressure points creates changes on two levels.

On the physical level, acupressure affects muscular tension, blood circulation, and other physiological functions. On a more subtle level, Traditional Chinese Medicine believes that acupressure, as well as acupuncture, helps to build the body's life energy to promote healing. When the normal flow of energy through the body is resumed, the body is believed to heal itself spontaneously.

Interestingly, a medical study using acupuncture for the treatment of menstrual cramps and pain was done by Dr. Joseph Helms, a family practitioner in Berkeley, California. In his study, 43 women were divided into four groups. All these women were using medication to control menstrual pain. One group of women received treatment with the acupuncture points necessary to control the menstrual pain symptoms. The other three groups received either false acupuncture treatment or no treatment. At the end of this 12-month study, 90 percent of those receiving real acupuncture treatment reported rapid and significant symptom relief. This included relief of cramping, nausea, back pain, headaches, and fluid retention. In contrast, only 36 percent of the women who received the false acupuncture treatments said that they noted symptom relief.

Other physicians using acupuncture and acupressure to treat endometriosis symptoms note similar results. Good results are more likely to occur in women with mild to moderate symptoms. Acupressure may not be as effective in women with more severe and advanced cases; these women may need to use Western medical treatments along with a variety of self-help therapies.

In any case, acupressure has much to offer the woman suffering from endometriosis. I suggest you try the following exercises to see if you find some that work for you.

Following the simple instructions, either you or a friend can stimulate the acupressure points through finger pressure. It is safe, painless, and does not require the use of needles. You can do this without the years of specialized training needed for the proper insertion of acupuncture needles.

How to Perform Acupressure

Acupressure should be done by yourself or by a friend, when you are relaxed. The room should be warm and quiet. Hands should be clean and nails trimmed to avoid bruising. If the hands are cold, warm them in water.

Work on the side of the body that has the most discomfort. If both sides are equally uncomfortable, choose whichever one you want. Working on one side seems to relieve the symptoms on both sides; energy or information appears to transfer from one side to the other.

Hold each indicated point with a steady pressure for 1 to 3 minutes. Apply pressure slowly with the tips or balls of the fingers. Make sure your hand is comfortable. Place several fingers over the area of the point. If you feel resistance or tension in the area to which you are applying pressure, you may want to push a little harder. However, if your hand starts to feel tense or tired, lighten the pressure a bit. Breathe gently while doing each exercise.

The acupressure point may feel somewhat tender. This means the energy pathway or meridian is blocked. During the treatment, the tenderness in the point should slowly go away. You may also have a subjective feeling of energy radiating from this point into the body. Many patients describe this sensation as very pleasant. Don't worry if you don't feel it—not everyone does. The main goal is relief from your symptoms.

To find the correct acupressure point, look in the photograph accompanying the exercise. Each point corresponds to specific points on the acupressure meridians. Massage the points once a day or more during the time that you have symptoms.

Exercise 1: Balances the Entire Reproductive System

This exercise is used to balance the energy of the female reproductive tract and alleviate all menstrual complaints. It also relieves pelvic and abdominal discomfort and low back pain, which are very common complaints in women with endometriosis.

Equipment: This exercise uses a knotted hand towel to put pressure on hard-to-reach areas of the back. Place the knotted towel on these points while your two hands are on other points. This increases your ability to unblock the energy pathways of your body.

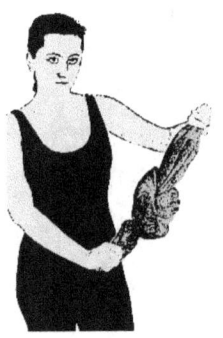 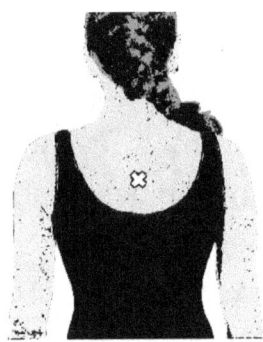

Lie on the floor with your knees up. As you lie down, place the towel between your shoulder blades on the spine. Hold each step for 1 to 3 minutes.

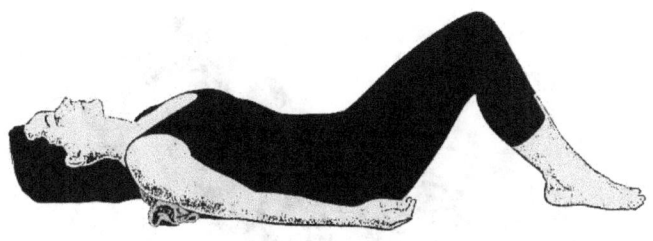

Cross your arms over your chest. Press your thumbs against the right and left inside upper arms.

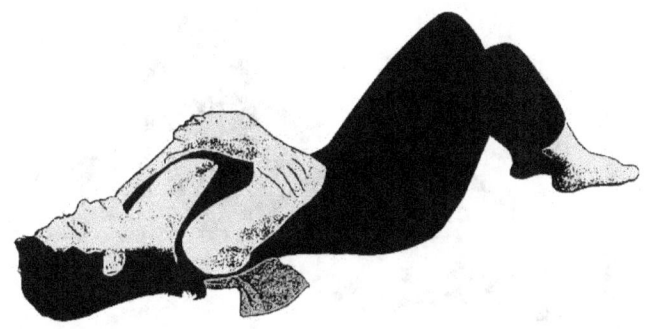

Left hand holds point at the base of the sternum (breastbone). Right hand holds point at the base of the head (at the junction of the spine and the skull).

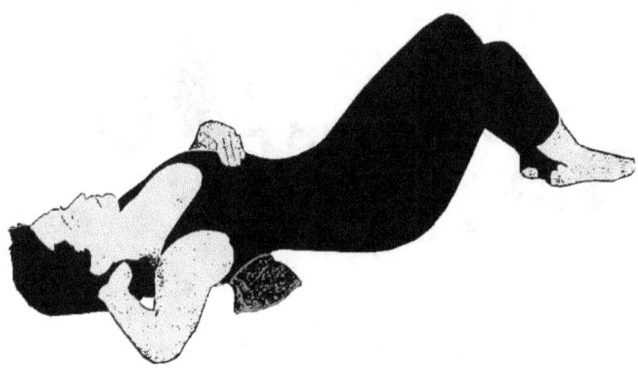

Interlace your fingers. Place them below your breasts. Fingertips should press directly against the body.

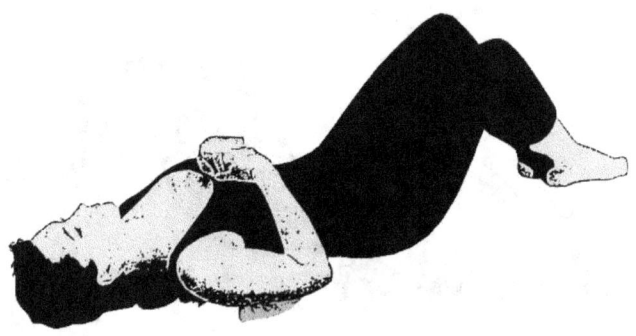

Move the knotted towel along the spine to the waistline.

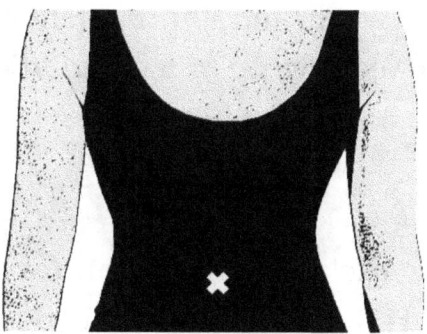

Left hand should be placed at the top of the pubic bone, pressing down. Right hand holds point on tailbone.

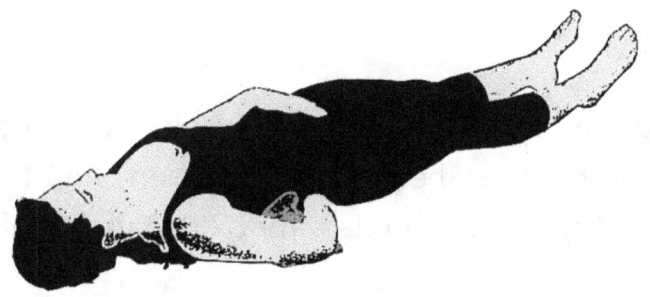

Exercise 2: Relieves Cramps, Bloating, Fluid Retention, Weight Gain

This sequence balances the points on the spleen meridian, used in acupressure to relieve menstrual cramps and pelvic and abdominal discomfort associated with endometriosis. Stimulation of these points also relieves premenstrual bloating and fluid retention and helps minimize weight gain in the period leading up to menstruation. The spleen meridian also helps regulate heavy menstrual bleeding.

Sit up and prop your back against a chair, or lie down and put your lower legs on a chair. Hold each step for 1 to 3 minutes.

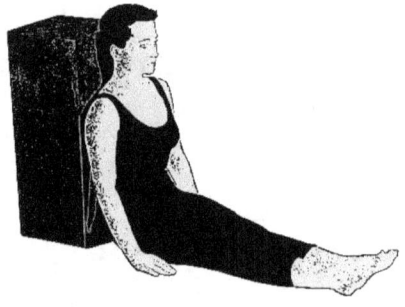

Left hand is placed in the crease of the groin where you bend your leg, one-third to one-half way between the hip bone and the outside edge of the pubic bone. Right hand holds a spot 2 to 3 inches above the knee.

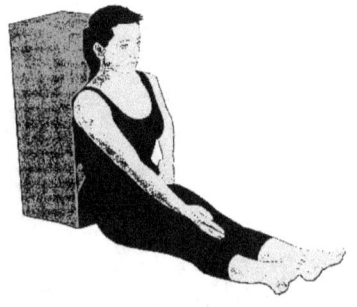

Left hand remains in the crease of the groin. Right hand holds point below inner knee. Follow the curve of the bone just below the knee. Hold the underside of the curve.

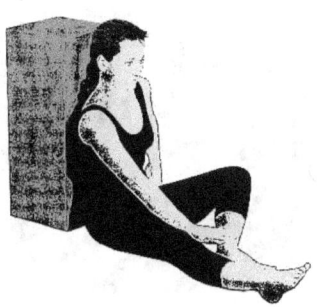

Left hand remains in the crease of the groin. Right hand holds the inside of the shin. To find this point, go four finger widths above the ankle bone. The point is just above the top finger.

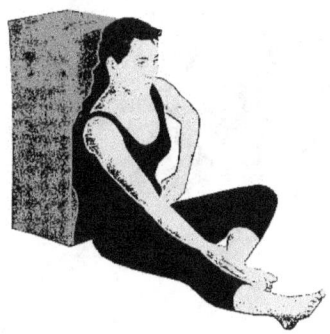

Left hand remains in the crease of the groin. Right hand holds the edge of the instep. To find the point, follow the big toe bone up until you hit a knobby, prominent small bone.

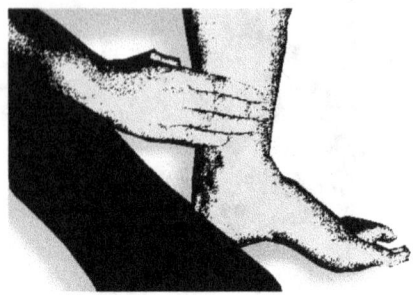

Left hand remains in the crease of the groin. Right hand holds the big toe over the nail, front and back of the toe.

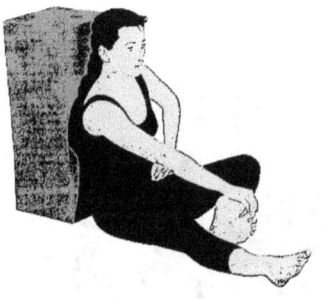

Exercise 3: Relieves Low Back Pain and Cramps

This exercise relieves menstrual cramps and low back pain by balancing points on the bladder meridian. This meridian relieves symptoms by balancing the energy of the female reproductive tract. These points are also used in Chinese medicine to relieve PMS symptoms, pelvic tension, and urinary problems, which often coexist with endometriosis.

Sit on the floor and prop your back against a wall or a heavy piece of furniture. Hold each step for 1 to 3 minutes.

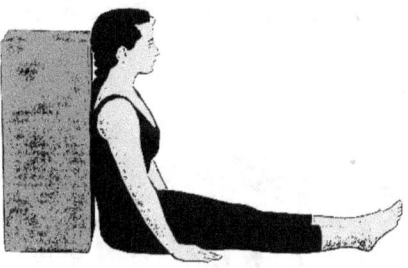

Alternative method: Lie on the floor and put your lower legs over the seat of a chair. Follow the exercise from that position.

Place left hand 1 inch above the waist on the muscle to the left side of the spine (muscle will feel firm and ropelike). Place right hand behind crease of the left knee.

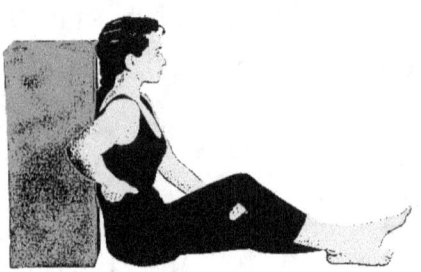

Left hand stays in the same position. Right hand is placed on the center of the back of the left calf. This is just below the fullest part of the calf.

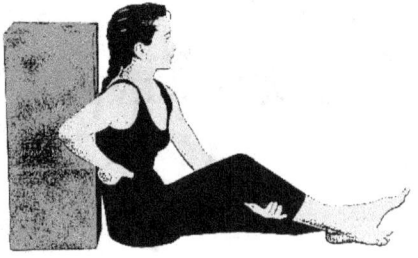

Left hand remains 1 inch above the waist on the muscle to the side of the spine. Right hand is placed just below the ankle bone on the outside of the left heel.

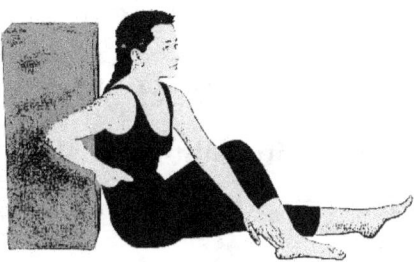

Left hand remains 1 inch above the waist on the muscle to the side of the spine. Right hand holds the front and back of the left little toe at the nail.

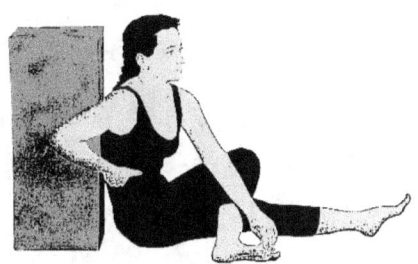

Exercise 4: Relieves Nausea

This exercise relieves the nausea and digestive symptoms that often occur with cramps and low back pain. Endometriosis can cause digestive symptoms when the implants invade the small intestine and colon.

Lie on the floor or sit up. Hold these points 1 to 3 minutes.

Left index finger is placed in navel and pointed slightly toward the head. Right hand holds point at the base of the head.

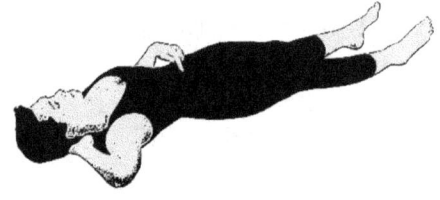

Exercise 5: Relieves Menstrual Fatigue and Stress

This sequence of points relieves the fatigue that women experience just prior to the onset of the menstrual period. For many women, tiredness may last through the first few days of menstruation. Women with heavy menstrual bleeding due to endometriosis may tire easily because of blood loss. This exercise can also relieve menstrual anxiety and depression, helpful to women suffering from significant stress in their lives. The second step in this sequence has traditionally been forbidden for use by pregnant women after their first trimester.

Sit up and prop your back against a chair. Hold each step for 1 to 3 minutes.

Left hand holds point at the base of the ball of the right foot. This point is located between the two pads of the foot.

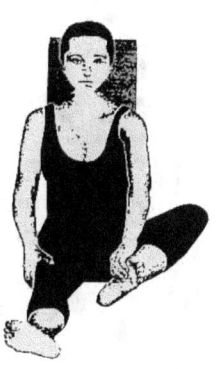

Left hand holds the point midway between the inside of the right anklebone and the Achilles tendon. The Achilles tendon is located at the back of the ankle.

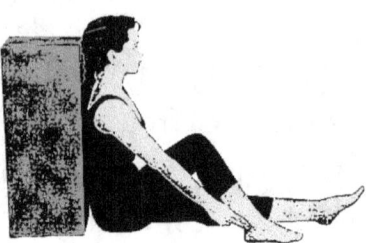

Left hand holds point below right knee. This point is located four finger-widths below the kneecap toward the outside of the shinbone. It is sensitive to the touch in many people.

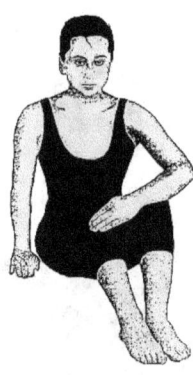

Exercise 6: Relieves Cramps, Digestive Symptoms, and Menstrual Irregularity

This exercise stimulates conception vessel points on the front of the body. These points help relieve the pain of menstrual cramps caused by endometriosis as well as constipation, which can accompany these problems. These points are also used to help treat menstrual irregularity.

Sit or lie in a comfortable position.

Place your fingertips on the point two finger-widths below the navel and hold.

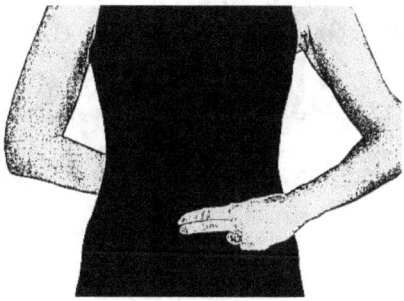

Move your fingertips to the point four finger-widths below the navel and hold.

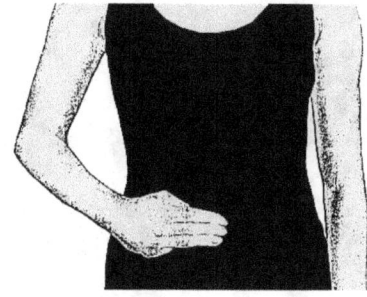

Exercise 7: Relieves Heavy Menstrual Bleeding

This sequence of points is important for the treatment of heavy menstrual flow, which can accompany endometriosis. Heavy menstrual bleeding is also a common cause of chronic fatigue and tiredness. This exercise involves the stimulation of points on the spleen meridian, which affect blood formation and menstrual problems.

Sit upright on a chair. Hold each step for 1 to 3 minutes.

Right hand holds point four finger-widths above the ankle bone.

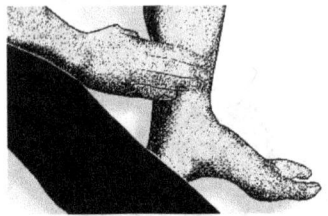

Right hand holds point above and below the nail of the big toe.

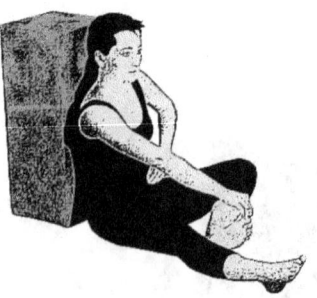

12

Treating Endometriosis with Drugs

Drugs and hormonal therapies have been the mainstay of the Western medical response to endometriosis for the past 30 to 40 years. A few of these medications are available to women over the counter, while other, stronger drugs need a doctor's prescription and careful monitoring is required.

Some medications—such as narcotics, birth control pills, male hormones and progestins, diuretics, and muscle relaxants—have been around for a long time and have been the traditional drug treatments for endometriosis. Others, specifically the prescription antiprostaglandins, synthetic male hormones, and GnRH (gonadotropin-releasing hormone) analogs, have been available for use in treating endometriosis in more recent years.

Medication can be very helpful in relieving endometriosis symptoms in the short run, but they are often accompanied by significant, and occasionally, even severe side effects. However, in the short term they can help to control the symptoms, if you can tolerate them well. In this chapter I discuss many of these medications.

Over-the-Counter Medications

Many women with endometriosis use over-the-counter pain and cramp medications because they mistakenly believe they are treating simple menstrual cramps. These products may provide some relief in the earliest stages of endometriosis, if symptoms are mild. As endometriosis progresses in severity, symptom relief from these drugs may not continue.

One of the oldest cramp-relief medications is simply aspirin. Interestingly, aspirin is a mild prostaglandin inhibitor, although it is only one-thirtieth as strong as the newer antiprostaglandin drugs. The F2 Alpha prostaglandins cause uterine contractions when present in the reproductive tract in high concentrations around the time of menstruation. In addition to worsening pain and cramps, these prostaglandins may accelerate the spread of endometriosis by causing retrograde menstruation.

Always take aspirin with food to avoid stomach discomfort and use it with great caution if you have a preexisting peptic ulcer or a tendency toward heartburn, because it can worsen or reactivate symptoms.

Another more modern prostaglandin inhibitor is ibuprofen. This drug is sold over the counter as Advil, Motrin or Nuprin, in 200 or 400 milligram dosages. The dose commonly used for menstrual pain and cramps is two tablets, or 400 milligrams, taken every six hours. Like aspirin, ibuprofen should be taken with food as it can cause gastrointestinal upset.

These medications are also available by prescription when taken in higher dosages. They include Motrin (in an 800 milligram dosage), Naprosyn or naproxen sodium as well as Ponstel. These drugs must be used carefully, however, since they can cause gastrointestinal bleeding and peptic ulcer disease or even reactivate a pre-existing ulcer.

Approximately 10 percent of women who use these medications report digestive symptoms, including heartburn, nausea, vomiting, diarrhea, constipation, and poor digestion. To lessen the likelihood of these side effects, always take these medications with food. Report any significant digestive symptoms to your physician. Some women report other unpleasant symptoms when using prostaglandin inhibitors—drowsiness, headaches, vertigo, dizziness, rashes, blurred vision, anemia, edema, and heart palpitations. Avoid using these drugs with aspirin, since both can cause gastrointestinal bleeding and irritation.

Some over-the-counter remedies for menstrual pain contain several drugs in combination. Products such as Midol, Pamprin, and a number of others contain aspirin, an antispasmodic to relieve muscle tension, caffeine (which causes widening in the diameter of peripheral blood vessels), and sometimes a diuretic for relief of congestive symptoms. Like the mild antiprostaglandins, they may be used frequently with early-stage, undiagnosed endometriosis.

Be careful to follow the dosage instructions on the bottle; if used in excess, many of these drugs can cause undesired side effects. Aspirin can cause gastric distress; caffeine can make people nervous and jittery and may also upset the stomach by increasing gastric acid secretion. Pamabrom, a diuretic agent used in several products, can lead to loss of minerals, like all diuretics. Another commonly used ingredient in these products is pyrilamine, an antihistamine.

Antihistamines are normally used to relieve symptoms of allergy-like nasal congestion. They also have the tendency to cause drowsiness or sedation and are used in menstrual remedies for these sedative effects. Although the doses used are small, some women who are sensitive may encounter side effects.

Prescription Medications

While certain types of medications for the relief of endometriosis are available over the counter (OTC), a number of drugs often used for this condition can only be prescribed by a physician. Medications are generally used to control moderate to severe symptoms.

Narcotics. Narcotics such as codeine are very effective painkillers and can certainly numb the discomfort of endometriosis or menstrual cramps. They do, however, have significant side effects and don't reverse the underlying cause of the menstrual cramps or halt the spread of endometrial implants. The side effects of narcotics commonly include constipation, nausea, and drowsiness. Be sure to avoid driving your car when using a narcotic painkiller because you may fall asleep at the wheel.

Other painkillers like Darvon or relaxants like Valium are also prescribed. Though Valium is an effective relaxant, it can also cause drowsiness and sedation. All of these drugs can be addictive. Women who use them on an ongoing basis often find that they need higher doses and more frequent usage in order to continue a beneficial therapeutic effect. I generally recommend that women use these drugs very infrequently and only if symptoms are particularly severe.

Birth Control Pills. These drugs have been the primary treatment for endometriosis since the 1950s. Many physicians still prescribe birth control pills as the treatment of choice for endometriosis. Birth control pills contain estrogen and a synthetic progesterone (or progestin) in varying doses. The estrogen and progestin in the birth control pills shut down your body's natural production of hormones. The hormones in the medication trick your pituitary and hypothalamus into thinking that your ovaries have produced high levels of hormones. As a result, the hypothalamus and pituitary stop secreting the hormones — FSH (follicle-stimulating hormone) and LH (luteinizing hormone) — that trigger ovarian function.

The pill also creates a state of pseudo-pregnancy, because it contains the same hormones found in high levels in women who are pregnant. The pills are given over a 12 month period to simulate the 9 months that women are pregnant and 3 months spent breastfeeding, which also suppresses normal menstrual cycles. This year long vacation from regular menstrual cycles can reduce endometriosis symptoms. Because the birth control pills prevent ovulation, they decrease the prostaglandin accumulation during the second half of the menstrual cycle. Prostaglandin accumulation has been linked to menstrual pain and cramps. The levels of estrogen and progestin in the birth control pills also cause lighter menstrual flow, a benefit for women with endometriosis who tend to have heavy bleeding and spotting.

The use of a low-estrogen-dose birth control pill is very important in order to reduce menstruation. The hormones used in the pill alter the endometrium (lining of the uterus) to create abnormal cells that do not cause pelvic implants, even if there is retrograde menstruation. Low-dose birth control pills currently contain less than 35 micrograms of estrogen. They are definitely preferred over high-dose estrogen pills, which can stimulate the growth of endometrial implants. As explained earlier, estrogen can trigger the acceleration and spread of endometrial growths. Thus, dosage is very important. It is important to understand that although low-dose pills can reduce pain and other symptoms of endometriosis, they do not eliminate the implants themselves.

Low-dose birth control pills are best used by young women in their teens and twenties who suffer from severe menstrual cramps and are at high risk of developing endometriosis. Other candidates for the birth control pill include women with diagnosed endometriosis who have just given birth and have not been on other previous therapy for endometriosis, such as the drug Danazol (discussed later in this chapter).

For these women, the oral contraceptive may help prevent the recurrence of endometriosis symptoms as well as prevent another pregnancy, if that is desired. Birth control pills can also be used by women who have had previous drug or surgical treatment for endometriosis, and don't wish to become pregnant. In all these cases, the birth control pill is used in the standard way: Women are given three weeks of hormones, taking one pill per day, followed by a week of rest with no hormonal intake.

Many women, however, should not take birth control pills as a treatment for endometriosis. These include women with a history of blood clots, high blood pressure, liver or gall bladder disease, pre-existing breast or uterine cancer, or those who smoke. Some women with milder cases of endometriosis find that their symptoms diminish with the use of the pill, but they experience uncomfortable side effects such as weight gain, fluid retention, breast tenderness, PMS mood changes, and headaches. In some cases, the side effects are so uncomfortable that the birth control pills must be discontinued.

Danazol. Danazol is used to treat endometriosis and fibrocystic breast disease. Marketed as Danocrine in the United States, it is a synthetic hormone derived from the male hormone testosterone. It induces a pseudo-menopause by directly depressing the output of FSH (follicle-stimulating hormone) and LH (luteinizing hormone) from the pituitary and lowering estrogen production by the ovaries. Because of this effect on the endocrine glands, Danazol is called a gonadotropin inhibitor.

Danazol also acts to alter the metabolism of estrogen and progesterone and to block the estrogen and progesterone receptors in the endometrial implants. These changes lead to both relief of endometriosis symptoms and shrinkage of the implants. Large masses and adhesions or scar tissue actually disappear. This offers tremendous benefit to women with endometriosis, 85 percent of whom report significant relief. Danazol may also cause the regression of fibrocystic breast lesions.

Treatment is generally instituted for 6 to 12 months, depending on the severity of the disease. Dosages range from 400 to 800 milligrams, in two daily doses, taken at night and during the day. The drug generally reduces estrogen to levels low enough to stop menstruation. Often this reduction takes several months.

Danazol does have drawbacks, however. For one thing, it does not cure endometriosis. One survey of 180 women conducted by the Endometriosis Association in Milwaukee, Wisconsin, reported that more than 50 percent of women surveyed who had taken Danazol either had no symptom relief or had a recurrence of symptoms immediately after stopping the drug. In another report in medical literature, 20 percent taking the drug noted a recurrence of endometrial symptoms within a year after stopping Danazol therapy. This incidence continues to increase with time.

Another problem that many women using Danazol encounter is unpleasant side effects. While Danazol itself does 't cause masculinization, it decreases estrogen levels enough that a woman's natural male hormonal response is accentuated. This can lead to acne, abnormal hair growth, increased oiliness of the skin or hair, weight gain, decrease in breast size, deepening of the voice, and even rarely, clitoral hypertrophy. These masculinizing effects are, unfortunately, not always reversible.

Due to the decline in the estrogen levels, women on Danazol may also have menopause symptoms such as hot flashes, night sweats, and vaginal dryness. Other unpleasant side effects include bloating, fluid retention, weight gain, changes in liver function, muscle cramps, headaches, dizziness, depression, and anxiety. Obviously, Danazol, for all its benefits, must be carefully monitored by a physician during the course of therapy.

GnRH Analogs. These drugs, such as Lupron and Nafarelin, have been tested experimentally in recent years as another treatment for endometriosis. They are chemically similar to the gonadotropin-releasing hormone (GnRH or LH-RH) that triggers secretion of LH and FSH by the pituitary. The pituitary in turn regulates the ovarian output of estrogen and progesterone. The analog drugs are given by nasal spray or injection and, like Danazol, inhibit the hypothalamus-pituitary-ovarian feedback loop. As a result, FSH and LH secretion is inhibited and estrogen levels decrease. Also like Danazol, these drugs produce relief of endometriosis and shrink endometrial implants. GnRH analogs have also been used for the treatment of other diseases for which suppression of estrogen is important, such as ovarian cysts.

One benefit of the GnRH analogs is that they don't have masculinizing side effects like Danazol. They do, however, produce the typical symptoms of menopause—hot flashes, mood swings, back and muscle pain, and headaches. They also increase the long-term risk of osteoporosis by lowering the estrogen level and increasing calcium excretion from the body. The side effects can be quite unpleasant; I have had a number of younger women see me in consultation purely to work with the menopausal side effects that the analogs cause.

Mirena Intrauterine Devices (IUD's). These IUD's are used for long-term birth control to prevent pregnancy. It is a T-shaped plastic frame that contains levonorgestrel, a synthetic progesterone, called a progestin. The Mirena IUD acts by thickening the cervical mucus to prevent sperm from reaching and fertilizing an egg.

The IUD is placed into the cervix or opening of the uterus through the vagina and the progestin is released locally into the uterine tissue. They are often used for women who want to prevent pregnancy and suffer from heavy bleeding due to endometriosis and other gynecological conditions. It has also been shown to be a helpful treatment for fibroid tumors, including providing relief of symptoms and even some reports of the tumors shrinking.

This IUD does, however, cause significant side effects for some women. Its insertion can cause severe pelvic or abdominal pain and cramping and even heavy and prolonged bleeding. In fact, several of my recent patients had to have the Mirena IUD removed right away because it caused excessive bleeding. It can also cause ovarian cysts, weight gain, headache, acne, breast tenderness, breakthrough bleeding, absence of periods and mood changes.

In summary, many drug therapies are available for treatment of endometriosis. Though many of these offer only symptomatic relief, certain drugs can shrink endometrial implants. Still, none of these therapies is curative and, in many cases, they cause unpleasant side effects. The stronger drugs must be prescribed and carefully monitored by a physician.

I always recommend that women on drug therapy for endometriosis also follow a complete all-natural treatment program to regulate and balance their hormonal levels, to build up their immune system to limit the spread of the tissue damage, and to control emotional stress. These self-help therapies, in combination with judicious use of medication, can provide effective relief for many women suffering from endometriosis.

Common Side Effects For:

Birth Control Pill
  Weight gain
  Fluid retention, bloating
  Breast tenderness
  Premenstrual syndrome
  Mood changes
  Headaches

GnRH Analogs
  Hot flashes, night sweats
  Vaginal atrophy
  Mood swings
  Increased calcium excretion
  Osteoporosis
  Breast tenderness
  High blood pressure
  Digestive changes
  Anemia
  Headaches, dizziness
  Increase in urinary frequency

Danazol
  Acne, oily hair and skin
  Abnormal hair growth
  Weight gain
  Decrease in breast size
  Deepening of the voice
  Clitoral hypertrophy
  Hot flashes, night sweats
  Vaginal atrophy
  Vaginitis
  Fluid retention, bloating
  Changes in liver function
  Muscle cramps
  Headaches, dizziness

Women with endometriosis should not use birth control pills if they have any of the following symptoms:

- Blood clots in the legs, pelvis, or lungs
- Fibroid tumors
- High blood pressure
- History of breast or uterine cancer
- Liver or gall bladder disease
- Use of cigarettes or tobacco products

Medications for Endometriosis

Over-the-Counter Medications
Aspirin
Ibuprofen (Advil, Nuprin)
Pamprin

Hormonal Therapies
Birth control pills
Natural progesterone
Danazol
Lupron
Nafarelin

Prescription Drugs
Antiprostaglandin Inhibitors
Motrin
Anaprox
Midol
Ponstel
Naprosyn

Narcotics
Codeine
Darvon

13

Surgery for Relief of Endometriosis

Many women with endometriosis never need surgery, primarily because these conditions are not causing severe physical symptoms. Many women with mild to moderate symptoms may handle the disease process quite effectively through a self-help program or drug and hormonal therapies. Remember that both problems may become less severe with the onset of menopause when the hormonal levels decrease. Endometriosis is stimulated by high levels of estrogen. Conservative management may allow a woman to preserve her uterus and avoid the physical and emotional stress of surgery. However, for some women with endometriosis, surgery is unavoidable and necessary. In this chapter I discuss the surgical techniques commonly used to treat these conditions, as well as their indications and risks.

Surgery for Endometriosis

With endometriosis, the goals of surgery are to relieve pain or to restore fertility and, ideally, prevent recurrence of the disease. Depending on the severity of the disease and the age of the patient, the physician may recommend either conservative surgery or more extensive surgery. Conservative surgery allows the preservation of the patient's reproductive organs while removing the endometriosis implants; more extensive surgery removes both the endometriosis implants and the reproductive organs.

Conservative Surgery. This involves the removal of the implants at the time the actual diagnosis is made by a laparoscopy. As discussed in Chapter 3, the laparoscope is an instrument that allows visualization of the pelvic cavity and the reproductive organs. Once the implants, adhesions, endometrial cysts, or other changes typical of endometriosis are visualized, treatment can be initiated at once. In many cases, this prevents the need for a second, follow-up surgical procedure after diagnosis.

Treatment consists of destroying the implants by the use of a laser or electrocautery. This technique can remove scarring or adhesions, implants, and small ovarian cysts.

Some physicians prefer laser therapy because it involves less blood loss, less thermal damage to the tissues by the instrument, and fewer postoperative adhesions. Also, cautery should be avoided in treating the fallopian tubes or bladder because of the risk of burning these tissues. However, in the hands of an experienced surgeon, cautery is also a very effective and useful technique. When faced with a choice, women should seek out physicians who are skilled at laparoscopic surgery. The doctor's technical proficiency in performing either technique is paramount in determining how good the results will be. To improve the cure rate, many physicians combine surgery with drug therapy like Danazol. Drug therapy is often given either pre- or postoperatively for a period of time to further reduce the risk of recurrence.

There are women for whom laparoscopic surgery is not a good option. Women with extensive endometriosis, many adhesions, involvement of the bowel or urinary tract, large endometrial cysts, or extensive disease in the ovaries may need more radical surgery. These problems are often beyond the scope of laser or cautery treatment and may require a larger incision and removal of the reproductive organs, as well as destruction of the implant and scar tissue.

However, some very experienced surgeons claim good treatment results even for women with severe endometriosis using laser therapy. This technique has even been used to restore fertility in women with severe adhesions and scar tissue with some success in promoting full term pregnancy.

How successful is conservative surgery? In those women who undergo surgery primarily to restore fertility, the success of the treatment depends on the extent of the disease process. Medical studies have shown that women with moderate endometriosis have a 50 to 60 percent pregnancy rate after surgery, while women with severe endometriosis have a 30 to 40 percent chance of conceiving.

The recurrence rate after surgery is fairly high. Studies have shown that the five-year recurrence rates are between 20 and 40 percent. Some women will eventually require a second laparoscopic procedure or even a total abdominal hysterectomy as treatment for recurrence.

Yet, given that laparoscopic surgery preserves the uterus and ovaries, I greatly prefer trying this route, if at all possible, rather than opting for the more drastic choice of hysterectomy. Even after menopause, our ovaries continue to produce female hormones that help to keep our tissues youthful and our bones and hearts healthy.

I have seen patients go under the knife and have hysterectomy and even ovariectomy and then suffer significant and unwanted complications. One of the worse outcomes is that some women will undergo a complete hysterectomy and then begin HRT only to find that their endometriosis was reactivated and their symptoms returned. These women feel trapped and cornered because they are much more depleted without their ovaries and now their treatment options are much less. It is worth taking the time and energy to research finding an experienced physician who can perform laparoscopic surgery rather than opting for hysterectomy, if at all possible.

Extensive Surgery. Surgeons often recommend more extensive surgery to women in their thirties and forties who have more severe disease and to women for whom fertility is not an issue. A woman in her thirties and forties who has completed or does not desire childbearing may elect to undergo major surgery, in which the surgeon opens the abdomen and removes the uterus and, unfortunately, even the ovaries along with all visible implants and adhesions.

To avoid an early menopause, the surgeon should try to spare the ovaries (or at least part of one ovary, if the endometriosis has attached itself to these glands) if at all possible. A premature surgical menopause can be difficult for women to tolerate when the ovaries are entirely removed. Symptoms such as hot flashes and vaginal dryness can be quite severe.

Also, the risk of developing osteoporosis over time is greater in these women.

As previously mentioned, there is a chance of reactivating the endometriosis in women who have had a total hysterectomy once they begin hormonal replacement therapy, because estrogen stimulates the growth of the implants. It may be impossible to remove all the microscopic implants during the operation, thus leaving behind tissue that can reactivate under hormonal stimulation. This can be a double-edged sword for younger women who don't want to suffer from hot flashes, yet are concerned about possible hormonal side effects. I have had patients who have been severely upset by this outcome, and understandably so.

Therefore, I strongly believe in preserving ovarian function if at all possible in women who must undergo surgery for endometriosis. Unfortunately, complete removal of the ovaries, tubes, and uterus is common, particularly if a woman is in her forties. This happens even when the disease is entirely treatable by removal of only the implants and scar tissue. I recommend that women choose their surgeon carefully, with the goal of preserving as many of their reproductive organs as possible without sacrificing the best therapeutic response. If major surgery is required, it is important to speak with several doctors to learn what options are available.

14

Putting Your Program Together

In this book, I have shared with you a complete self-care program to help prevent and relieve your symptoms of endometriosis. I recommend trying the treatment options that feel most comfortable to you. You may find that certain exercise routines or stress reduction techniques feel better to you than others. If that is the case, practice the ones that bring the greatest sense of relief for your particular symptoms.

Always keep in mind that your ultimate goal is relief of your endometriosis symptoms and a great improvement in your overall health and well-being. I usually recommend beginning any self-care program slowly while you get used to the changes in lifestyle. People differ in their ability to adjust to major lifestyle changes. Though some of my patients like to eliminate their old, unhealthy habits as quickly as possible, many other women find such rapid changes in long-term habits too stressful. Find the pace that works for you.

Enjoy the program. I always tell my patients to regard their self-care program as an enjoyable adventure. The exercises and stress-reduction techniques should give you a sense of energy and well-being. The menus and food selections I've recommended in this book provide you with an opportunity to try delicious and healthful new recipes and meal plans.

As you do the program, don't set up unrealistic or overly strict expectations for yourself. You don't have to be perfect to get great results. Just follow the guidelines of the program as best you can and as your schedule permits.

It is not a major issue if you forget to take your vitamins occasionally or don't have time to exercise on a particular day. Don't be discouraged if you can't follow the dietary recommendations on vacations, holidays, and birthdays. Periodically review the guidelines outlined in this book and continue to adapt your lifestyle to the healthful suggestions that I've shared with you from my years of medical practice. Over time you will notice many beneficial changes.

Be your own feedback system. Your body will tell you if you are on the right track and if what you are doing is making you feel better. It will also tell you if your current diet and emotional stresses are worsening your symptoms. Remember that even moderate changes in your habits can make significant differences.

The Endometriosis Workbook

Fill out the workbook section of this book. The workbook questionnaires will help you determine which areas in your life have contributed the most to your symptoms and need the most improvement. Review the workbook every month or two as you follow the self-help program. The workbook will help you see the areas in which you are making the most progress, with both symptom relief and the adoption of healthier lifestyle habits. The workbook can help give you feedback in an organized and easy-to-use manner.

Diet and Nutritional Supplements

I recommend that you make all nutritional changes gradually. Many women find breakfast the easiest meal to change because it is simple and often eaten at home. To change your other meals and snacks, periodically review the list of foods to eliminate and foods to emphasize. Each month, pick a few foods that you are willing to eliminate from your diet. Try in their place the foods that help prevent and relieve endometriosis symptoms. The recipes and menus in Chapter 5 should be very helpful; use the meal plans as helpful guidelines while you restructure your diet to suit your needs.

Vitamins, minerals, essential fatty acids, and herbal supplements can help complete your nutritional needs and speed up the healing process. I have found the use of these nutritional supplements to be a very beneficial, even essential, part of your program.

Stress-Reduction and Breathing Exercises

The stress-reduction and breathing exercises play an important role in facilitating the physical healing process. I find that all my patients heal more rapidly from almost any problem when they are calm, happy, and relaxed. The visualization exercises can help you set a blueprint in your mind for optimal health; this enables your body and mind to work together in harmony.

Begin the program by putting aside 10 to 15 minutes each day, depending on the flexibility of your schedule. Try the stress-reduction and breathing exercises listed in this book that you feel most drawn towards. Choose the combination that works best for you. Practice stress management on a regular basis and be aware of your habitual breathing patterns. Both techniques will help normalize your hormonal balance, relax your uterine, pelvic, and back muscles, and release tension, giving you a more comfortable menstrual period.

You do not need to spend enormous amounts of time on these exercises. Many women are too busy, for example, to spend an hour a day meditating. Even 10 minutes out of your daily schedule can be helpful. You may find that the quietest times for you are early in the morning before you get out of bed or late at night before going to sleep. Some women simply choose to take a break during the day. You can close the door to your office or go into your bedroom at home for 10 to 15 minutes to relax. Use the time to breathe deeply, do the visualizations, or meditate. You will be much calmer and more relaxed afterward.

Physical Exercise, Stretches, and Acupressure

I recommend that you do moderate exercise on a regular basis, at least three times a week. Aerobic exercise can improve both circulation and oxygenation to tight, constricted muscles of your entire body, including your pelvic area, thereby helping you relax. It is important, however, to do your exercise routine slowly and comfortably. Frenetic exercise that is too fast-paced can push your muscles to the point of exhaustion and tense them further. Women with endometriosis-related pain and cramps need to keep their muscles and joints flexible and supple. To this end, try the fitness and flexibility exercises in this book.

To do the stretches and acupressure massage, set aside a half-hour each day for the first week or two of your self-help program. Try the exercises that appeal to you. After an initial period of exploration, choose the ones that you enjoy the most and that seem to give you the most relief. Practice them on a regular basis so that they can help to prevent and reduce your symptoms.

Conclusion

I want to inspire you that you have a tremendous ability to heal and can enjoy radiant female health and well-being. By having access to the information, education, and health resources contained in this book, you can play a major role in creating your own state of great health. Practice the beneficial self-care techniques that I've outlined in this book. Follow good nutritional habits, exercise, and practice stress-reduction techniques regularly.

By combining these beneficial principles of self-care, you can enjoy the same wonderful results that my patients and I have had in restoring your female health and hormonal balance.

Love,

Dr. Susan

About Susan Richards, M.D.

Dr. Susan Richards is one of the foremost authorities in the fields of family medicine and alternative medicine. Dr. Richards has successfully treated many thousands of patients emphasizing alternative health and integrative medicine in her clinical practice. Her mission is to provide her patients with safe and effective alternative therapies to greatly enhance their health and well-being.

A graduate of Northwestern University Feinberg School of Medicine, she has served on the clinical faculty of Stanford University School of Medicine and taught in their Division of Family and Community Medicine.

Her Facebook page, Dr. Susan's Healthy Living, has over one million followers. She is also an ordained minister and her ministry receives over a million prayer requests for healing each year.

Notes

Notes

Notes

References

Brown CS, Ling FW, Wan JY, et al. Efficacy of static magnetic field therapy in chronic pelvic pain: A double-blind pilot study. Am J Obstet Gynecol. 2002;187:1581–1587.

Brown CS, Parker N, Ling F, et al. Effect of magnets on chronic pelvic pain. Obstet Gynecol. 2000;95:S29.

Cai XS, et al., 43 cases of endometriosis treated by differentiation of syndromes, Shanghai Journal of Traditional Chinese Medicine 1982; 4: 12-13

Cao LX, Endometriosis as treated by traditional Chinese medicine, Journal of the American College of Traditional Chinese Medicine 1983; 1:54-57

Chang HM (ed.), Abstracts of Chinese Medicine, 1986-present, Chinese Medicinal Materials Research Centre, Shatin, Hong Kong.

Covens AL, Christopher P, Casper RF. The effect of dietary supplementation with fish oil fatty acids on surgically induced endometriosis in the rabbit. Fertil Steril. 1988;49:698–703.

Dai DY, 30 cases of endometriosis treated by taking Chinese herbs orally, externally, and by enema, Shanghai College of Traditional Chinese Medicine 1982; 3:34-35.

Han ML, Treatment of endometriosis with gossypol, in Recent Advances in Chinese Herbal Drugs (Zhou JH and Liu GZ, eds.), 1991 Science Press, Beijing.

Hardy, Mary L. "Herbs of Special Interest to Women." Journal of the American Pharmaceutical Association. March/April, 2000. 40(2): pp. 234-242.

He XL and Frosolone S, The treatment of endometriosis with traditional Chinese medicine, Journal of the American College of Traditional Chinese Medicine 1989; 7(1-2):31-48.

Hu GZ and Li XY, 48 endometriosis patients treated by the principle of eliminating stagnation and activating blood circulation, Shanghai Journal of Traditional Chinese Medicine 1995; 2: 38-40.

Jiang JN, et al., Clinical observation of 64 cases of endometriosis treated by blood vitalizing and stagnation-eliminating therapy, ACTA Chinese Medicine and Pharmacology 1992; 1:38-39.

Jin JL, 45 cases of endometriosis treated by blood circulation promoting and stasis removing therapy and laboratory analysis for nail-fold microcirculation, Shanxi Journal of Traditional Chinese Medicine, 1990; 11(9): 402-403.

Jin YC, Teaching rounds: endometriosis, International Journal of Oriental Medicine 1992; 17(4): 1206-210.

Li XY, Method of kidney tonifying and stasis removing for 74 cases of endometriosis, Shanghai Journal of Traditional Chinese Medicine, 1991; 7:20-21.

Lin YH, et al., Analysis of 85 cases of endometriosis treated by integrating traditional and Western medicine, Zhejiang Journal of Traditional Chinese Medicine 1989; 24(4): 159-160.

Lin YQ, et al., An approach to treatment of endometriosis by traditional Chinese medicine, Fujian Journal of Traditional Chinese Medicine 1988; 19(6): 21-23.

Liu DF, et al., A mechanism approach and clinical observation on endometriosis treated by therapy of promoting blood circulation and removing stasis, Chinese Journal of Integrated Traditional and Western Medicine 1983; 3(4): 207-209.

Liu Jian, Li Xiangyun, and Hu Xiaomei, Clinical observation on patients with endometriosis treated by tonifying kidney and removing blood stasis, Chinese Journal of Integrated Traditional and Western Medicine, 1998; 4(3): 166-169.

Noble-JG et al. "The Effects of Interferential Therapy Upon Cutaneous Blood Flow in Humans." Clinical Physiology. January, 2000. 20(1): pp.2-7.

Qu JZ and Liu GZ, Wen Hua Yin combined with ear-pressing therapy for the treatment of 54 cases of endometriosis, Shanxi Journal of Traditional Chinese Medicine 1992; 13 (5): 198-199.

Shao GQ, et al., Clinical and experimental research on 156 cases of endometriosis treated by therapy of promoting blood circulation and removing stasis, Shanghai Journal of Traditional Chinese Medicine 1980; 3:4-6

Tang BJ, Traditional Chinese herbal and acupuncture treatment for female infertility (part II), International Journal of Oriental Medicine 1991; 16(3): 151-161.

Wang DZ, Wang ZQ and Zhang ZF, Study on the treatment of endometriosis with removing blood-stasis and purgation method, Chinese Journal of Integrated Traditional and Western Medicine 1991; 11(9): 524-526.

Wang Qi and Dong Zhilin, Modern Clinical Necessities for Traditional Chinese Medicine, 1990 China Ocean Press, Beijing.

Wang ZQ, Zhang ZF, and Wang DZ, Clinical and experimental studies of stasis-reducing and viscus-opening therapy for endometriosis, Shanghai Journal of Traditional Chinese Medicine 1992; 9: 8-12.

Yang Yifan, Chinese Herbal Medicines: Comparisons and Characteristics, 2002 Churchill Livingstone, London.

Yano Y. Effect of dietary supplementation with eicosapentaenoic acid on surgically induced endometriosis in the rabbit. Nippon Sanka Fujinka Gakkai Zasshi. 1992;44:282–288.

Yu CQ, Effect of Nei Yi Fang on plasma endorphin levels during the menstrual cycle in women with endometriosis, Chinese Journal of Integrated Traditional and Western Medicine, 1995; 15(1): 6-8.

Yu CQ, Influence of Nei Yi Wan #2 on levels of beta-EP and DynA in endometriosis, Chinese Journal of Integrated Traditional and Western Medicine 1993; 13(1): 7-9.

Zhuang B and Xia GC, Correlation between treatment of syndrome differentiation and basic body temperature in 21 cases of endometriosis, Shanxi Journal of Traditional Chinese Medicine 1990; 11(12): 537.

Huang Bingshan and Wang Yuxia, Thousand Formulas and Thousand Herbs of Traditional Chinese Medicine, vol. 2, 1993 Heilongjiang Education Press, Harbin.

Yan Jingxi and Pan Guodong, Review of pharmacology studies and applications of Xuefu Zhuyu Tang, Journal of the Shandong College of Traditional Chinese Medicine 1993; 17(6): 423-425.

State Administration of Traditional Chinese Medicine, Advanced Textbook on Traditional Chinese Medicine and Pharmacology, (vol. 2) 1995-6 New World Press, Beijing.

www.ingramcontent.com/pod-product-compliance
Lightning Source LLC
Chambersburg PA
CBHW081059290526
45795CB00006B/1921